Soul Letters for the Cancer Sojourner

© Jo Hilder 2013

Copyright Notice

SOUL LETTERS FOR THE CANCER SOJOURNER

© 2013 Jo Hilder. All rights reserved.

ISBN # 978-0-9873681-6-4

This manuscript is protected by copyright. No part of this book may be reproduced, stored in a retrieval system, or transmitted in any form or by any means electronic, mechanical, photocopying, recording or otherwise without the prior permission of the author/publisher.

All rights reserved worldwide.

Acknowledgements

For Carolyn, who was there for me right in the middle of it all, and continues to be there for me no matter what – friend, coach, inspiration and co-conspirator in joy, mayhem and imagination.

Thank you to Abigail Westbrook again for the fabulous cover artwork.

Thank you also to my loyal and relentless tribe of supporters, particularly Anita Tang, Daniel Turner, Brad Fitzpatrick, Sue Anderson-Stevens, Janine Pace, Georgia Thomas, Fiona Crain, Sallie-Ann and Paul Macklin, Mark and Michelle Falzon, Candy Burls, Tammie Ison, Jenni and Darryl Shaw and Emma Gilbert.

To my wonderful Ben, thank you.

And to you, dear reader, for opening your heart and allowing me in, thank you.

Table of Contents

Introduction	7
Chapter 1 - This is the beginning	16
Chapter 2 - Choose our own cancer adventure	24
Chapter 3 - You Can Change One Thing Today	30
Chapter 4 - Cancer Never Wins.	34
Chapter 5 - My Name Is Not Cancer	36
Chapter 6 - Letting Others Be Part Of Your Story When You Have Cancer	42
Chapter 7 - When 'Support' Means Something Different For Everybody	45
Chapter 8 - Finding Out The Deep Meaning Behind Your Having Cancer	50
Chapter 9 - Some Negative Thoughts About Positive Thinking	53
Chapter 10 - Telling Yourself The Truth	60
Chapter 11 - You're Okay	66
Chapter 12 - Not My Time	71
Chapter 13 - Creativity And Cancer	74
Chapter 14 - How To Be An Inspiration	81
Chapter 15 - Your Story Matters	85
Chapter 16 - Your Wonderful, Powerful, Imperfect Story	88
Chapter 17 - Your Burning, Broken, Beautiful Story	93
Chapter 18 - Cancer Winners and Losers, Fighters and Survivors	98
Chapter 19 - We Feel It All	103
Chapter 20 - Make Cancer Pay	108
Chapter 21 - Curing "Burnt Toast" Syndrome	113

Chapter 22 - You're Going To Make It   **116**

Chapter 23 - No More Dramas   **119**

Chapter 24 - Funny Things People Say When You Have Cancer   **122**

Chapter 25 - When Dignity Wears A Size Smaller   **126**

Chapter 26 - Buy A Ticket   **132**

Chapter 27 - What Really Matters   **137**

Chapter 28 - Believe What God Says About You   **141**

Chapter 29 - Big Far Away, Where Hope Waits For Me   **146**

Chapter 30 - The Three Questions   **151**

Epilogue   **157**

Introduction

In July 2003, after several months of feeling unwell and being virtually ignored by my doctor, I was diagnosed with stage 3B Non-Hodgkin's lymphoma. A CT scan revealed the tumor in my chest was almost as big a saucer. My diagnosis saw me literally thrown into another world hundreds of kilometers away from my husband and four young children as I began an aggressive regime of chemotherapy and radiotherapy lasting six months. Thank God the treatment was successful in curing me of cancer, but if I'd thought chemotherapy and radiotherapy could fix all the problems cancer brought along with it, boy, did I have another thing coming.

The biggest lesson I learned from having cancer is there's more than one way for the damn thing to kill you.

The worst impacts cancer had on my life had nothing to do with the actual lymphoma, the side effects of treatment, or the duration of the illness. Over those months, I saw and learned things I'd never be able to unsee or unlearn. I was more afraid, confused, in pain, depressed and lonely than ever before in my life. Others perceived and treated me differently because of cancer, and I'd perceived and treated them differently right back again. I found out cancer is far more than just a disease – it's a place, with a language, geography and a culture all its own. Being diagnosed with cancer is winning a like a role in a play you didn't audition for, a drama complete with a script, stage directions, and even a special wardrobe to wear.

And I totally sucked at it.

By early 2004 my hair was growing back, I'd regained the weight I lost (dammit), and even resumed work. But despite the return of my energy and appetite, I still felt I wasn't back to normal. In fact, I had no idea what normal even was anymore. Post-cancer, my world and everyone in it looked completely different. My thoughts and beliefs about the kinds of things that can happen to people - even when they live good lives and do all the "right" things - had changed. I still had no idea what I'd done or hadn't done to make cancer happen to me, so was baffled as to what changes I should make to stop it coming back. And most upsettingly, despite having been told with annoying frequency what didn't kill me would make me stronger, I'd developed a nasty anxiety disorder, and was referred to see a psychologist.

Cancer did more to me than just make me physically sick - it was a catalyst for the emergence of all kinds of thoughts and beliefs I didn't even realize I had. For example, my faith tradition dictated cancer was a kind of lesson I was supposed to learn, but no matter how I tried, I simply couldn't make sense of it the way others seemed to expect me to. My life was great before cancer. I was great before cancer. Exactly what kind of God would teach me something through such terrible means? Further, people expected me to be able to interpret my experience for them, providing them with a kind of moral to the story. I just couldn't. I hadn't been positively transformed by having cancer, and neither had my family. In fact, my husband suffered the most shocking depression, and several years after I regained my health, was admitted to a residential rehab facility to deal with his alcoholism.

People assumed I'd won some kind of battle against cancer simply because I didn't die, but I didn't feel as though I'd fought, and I certainly didn't feel like a winner afterwards. In fact, no one actually seemed to know what "fighting" cancer even meant - was it mental, spiritual, or just something they said to people with cancer to make them feel less redundant and useless? Most of the people I'd met when I had cancer simply sat around and accepted whatever others wanted to do to them to make cancer go away, myself included. The idea of "fighting cancer" seemed abstract and even violent, particularly when talking about a vulnerable, sick body needing careful care and nurture. As ambivalent as I was about what fighting cancer meant to me, I felt compelled to involve myself in real and tangible ways to repel cancer and keep it away. Throwing myself into volunteering and fundraising for cancer charities, I commenced a bitter campaign against cancer and all it represented, to me, and to the people I loved - disempowerment, pain, failure and an overwhelming sense of loss and grief over lost and thwarted hopes and dreams.

And then, something happened. As I helped raise money for cancer research and support, and began to speak to others about my experience both during and after cancer, my story began to have a meaning. Rather than being a liability or a failure, my having cancer had become a skill set. I started to see how my experience could help other people. Calling on the communications skills I'd developed over the years and my experience as a cancer patient, I began speaking up and advocating for others, helping improve cancer services and access to treatment for people living in remote areas. I trained as a support group leader, and studied health promotion at university. I then went on to work for a cancer charity, organizing fundraising events and coordinating prevention programs. It was whilst running support and survivorship groups I began to confirm for myself the intrinsic power of story – the positive and empowering impact someone can have on another simply by sharing their cancer experience - the real one, not the one we think others want to hear. I realized we'd all been doing an awful lot of telling people with cancer what to think, feel and believe about cancer and how to experience it, but not a lot of reporting back from the front line about what it was really like. There were an awful lot of people not subscribing to the cancer battle cliché, and not giving cancer the power to define them - amazing, imperfect people facing death with grace and acceptance, incredible people living with cancer and not being victims or heroes, wonderful folks who refused to give cancer the power to change them, for better or for worse. I decided it was time to begin some new conversations about cancer - conversations which didn't include redundant clichés and platitudes, which helped people with cancer see they were always better and stronger and more interesting than cancer, empowering them to define their own cancer experience. And importantly, conversations which never included a post-script about someone "losing their battle with cancer" - not because they didn't die, but because cancer was never, ever able to beat them.

There are an awful lotta books about cancer out there, and this is my second contribution to this conversation. My first, Things Not To Say To Someone Who Has Cancer, is a practical guide of what to say and do when someone you love or know is diagnosed other than the usual cliché's - a book I wish had been around when I was sick. The book you're holding now is the other one I wished I'd had back then. I didn't want to read a book about cancer resembling a "with deepest sympathy" greeting card. I also didn't want to read books about cancer curing diets, or about how my negative thinking caused cancer. Other people's amazing personal transformation cancer stories made me feel like a dummy, because

I couldn't make head or tail of my own journey. I just wanted someone to tell me "What you're feeling is absolutely normal, and neither good nor bad. Others have been where you are now. Being scared, whiny and less than heroic is absolutely permitted. Talking about your anger and confusion will not make cancer worse. You can absolutely be trusted to decide what's best for you. Whatever happens – whatever happens - everything is going to be okay".

Maybe I just haven't found that book yet. Or maybe I was meant to write it.

This collection of letters is written straight from my cancer sojourners soul to yours. Each one comes from a place of experience, questioning and reflection, yet also from a place of practicality and pragmatism. You won't find anything ephemeral or airy-fairy here – this is stuff I learned the hard way, and some of it I'm still navigating and exploring. I offer no firm solutions or formulas for "success", no paths for spiritual transcendence or guarantees of survival in the face of cancer – just a comforting hand on your shoulder, and a voice which says, perhaps a little tremblingly, but always with total honesty, "I know. Me too."

I vividly remember what it's like to be inside a body people talk about as if it wasn't inhabited by a wonderful, beautiful and intelligent mind, heart and soul. I know what it's like to be addressed as the thing you hate most, and would be rid of in a hot minute if you only knew how – the tumor, the metastases, the cancer, the stage 3B diffused B-cell Non-Hodgkin's lymphoma. I know what it's like to look into people's eyes and see a movie of your funeral playing there. I know what its like to lose hope you'll ever see your children grow up, or survive long enough to see your husband once again gloriously consumed with just little, trivial things. I know what it's like to have your imagination, once occupied with making amazing things and making amazing things happen, slowly but surely possessed by panic and anxiety. I know what its like to be trapped mentally and emotionally in a perpetual cycle of prophesying catastrophes over yourself, catastrophes you've come to believe are rational possibilities. I know, really, I do.

While nothing anyone says can make those things go away, I'd like to walk this part of your life with you. Soul Letters is my love note to you - many love notes in fact. I don't want to surround you with pseudo-spiritual fluff-balls, or cover your eyes and give you something to bite on until it's all over. I just want to sit and agree with you – yes, you bet, this thing is crappy and unfair, and just plain old hard. Nobody wants to go through it, but go through it we must. Cancer is awful, but this isn't your fault. You have not failed - yourself, or anyone else. This is what I know - regardless of how weak, confused and helpless you find yourself right now, you're still better, stronger, and always much, much more than cancer.

Each of the chapters in Soul Letters has appeared as a blog post on my website at www.johilder.com under the category Soul Letters For The Cancer Sojourner. I invite you to visit the posts and leave comments and feedback. I read every single comment you leave there, and look forward to knowing your thoughts and experiences with cancer, or on the topics I cover in Soul Letters. I'd love to hear from you, receive your feedback on the book, and know your story. You can contact me via my website at www.johilder.com

Love, Jo

Chapter 1
This Is The Beginning.

This is the beginning.

I know what you're going to say. I've just been diagnosed with cancer – how can you say this is the beginning?

I know a cancer diagnosis feels nothing like a beginning.

It feels like a door just slammed shut.

It feels like all your dreams for the future were just cancelled.

It feels like being put off a train at a station in a place not particularly pleasant or interesting, while everyone else gets to stay on the train and keep going somewhere lovely and exciting. And you don't know if the train will ever be back for you.

Cancer feels like the end of something. The end of everything.

Or just the end - full stop.

And you're right - it is the end.

It's the end of the part of your life before this one.

It's the end of the way things used to be.

It's the end of – well, let's face it, God knows what. And that's the frustration, isn't it? You know it's the end of something, but you can't possibly know all the ways just yet. All you do know is what you hope it isn't the end of.

There's another thing cancer is the end of – it's the end of never speaking the unspeakable.

Cancer certainly is the end of some things. It's the end of pretending these kinds of things don't happen to us, to me. It's the end of thinking you have plenty of time to travel, to change, to forgive or put it right. Cancer is the end of believing it doesn't matter how you treat your body, your body will always bounce back.

Cancer can also be the end of thinking your body *is* you.

Your body may have cancer, but you are not merely what constitutes your body. Your body is just one part of you. There are other parts of you cancer cannot reach, and those parts may be about to come into their own.

Cancer can feel like the end of you being the boss of you, or knowing where you're going in life, of self-determination and control and autonomy. It can feel as though you've been forced into a process of personal transformation you weren't ready for, and didn't ask for, when you thought you and everything else was perfectly okay before cancer came along, thank you very much.

When it comes to cancer, there may be a few things you lose an element of control over. But here's something I'd like to share with you - the personal transformation part of cancer is totally optional. If you choose not to give cancer the power to improve you, just as I'm sure you've no wish to give cancer the power to lessen you, then good for you. But I'd also like to tell you what I've learned about cancer – it changes things. It can change the way you see the world, or your perceptions about the kinds of things that can happen to people. Cancer may change your body, or force you to have it changed in order to make cancer go away, and this can feel unfair, because it is. Cancer may increase your sense of fear, or your capacity for courage. Cancer changes things, and sometimes the thing it changes is *us*.

Some of the things cancer changes can't be changed back to the way they were before, and this can be cause for anger, grief and sorrow. But sometimes the change is exactly what you wanted or needed to happen. You may feel some of the things cancer changes had to change anyway, and it's about time. However, many more people feel cheated by cancer than feel this way. Being made to change by a force you can't control can make you angry, and many people stubbornly defy the changes – physical, emotional or spiritual - cancer forces upon them. But there are some kinds of change that can put you ahead of cancer, and help you feel on top of it instead of underneath it. Every time we make or allow a change, it's a new beginning, and with new beginnings come endings too. You may be angry and feel cheated. You may experience resentment and resistance. But the choice about how much of the change cancer brings you welcome or accept always remains with you.

This is the beginning - the beginning of your cancer journey.

Think of one of those roadside maps, the ones with the big arrow pointing to an "X" which says, "you are here".

Well, you are here.

And in order to go forward - and not simply sit down in the road and wait for something to happen to you, or for someone to make it happen - those of us who make this particular journey must simply pull on some boots and get started.

Perhaps everything you thought was sure and certain is falling apart and coming undone, and all you see are walls closing in around you. Perhaps this is the darkest time you've ever faced in your life. Please know that despite what's happening in your world, what it may feel like to you and where your future may seem to be heading, this is not the end.

I've been where you are now, and I'm here to tell you my story. You'll have the opportunity to tell yours as well. Above all else, please know - your story matters. It matters to me, and I'm not the only one it matters to.

You may think you need to be concerned about where exactly you're going and how on earth you'll get there and all the things which might happen along the way, but at the moment, you don't need to worry about those things What's important is starting - and here you are, just about to do it. The road is stretched out before you, and what was is now behind you. You may never have the opportunity to begin again like this, and you know what? That's exactly what's happening. Regardless of what lies ahead, and how long you'll be journeying for - with or without cancer - you're beginning again.

This is the beginning.

To see this as a beginning, you may have to use your imagination a little. Everything you think you know about cancer could be telling you all kinds of things about how this is likely to go. Our memory and our history are there to protect us from danger, to keep us safe from harm, but your memory and history aren't going to help you this time. What you think you know about cancer doesn't have anything good to say about this, so it may be best if you start with an open mind. You need something only your imagination can give you, and that's hope.

Hope is living out of your imagination instead of from your memory and your history.

You have the opportunity right now to begin living from your imagination, instead of from your history.

You can begin to change what you think you know about yourself, about having cancer, about the others and your life and the way things are in the world. You have a chance to change your mind, and even to change your self.

Many people never get a chance to do this. And here you are with exactly this opportunity.

Look up. There's the map telling you where you are. Look down. There are your boots, and it's time to set off.

Dear friend; here's what I really want you to know, and what I'll be here to remind you of for the next thirty letters as we journey together. Despite what you may have thought about what it means to have cancer, and despite where this road leads, and how long you journey for from here on in, this is not the end.

This is the beginning.

Chapter 2

Choose Your Own Cancer Adventure.

Everyone's experience of cancer is different, except for the parts which seem almost universal.

One thing I've noticed which is almost the same for everyone diagnosed with cancer is the widespread perception amongst the people around them there has to be a moral to a cancer story. You know - a point, a lesson or a conclusion to be drawn from it.

I think there's two reasons we feel it's so important to have an answer to cancer -

1) We believe everything that happens in life is there to teach us something.

2) We want to believe everything has a positive side, if we choose to see it.

When it comes to cancer, both these can certainly be true. For some, attaching a sense of purpose can give cancer some kind of meaning, and God knows, sometimes we need to feel there's a meaning, otherwise we'd need a psychologist as well as an oncologist. In fact, many do.

But a lot of people with cancer don't want to see a deeper meaning in it. For them, cancer isn't the most amazing or interesting thing which ever happened to them. Further, a lot of folks don't want to be changed or defined by cancer.

After a cancer diagnosis - ours or someone else's - we may (naturally) feel shocked, confused and upset. Sometimes a sense of ongoing, subversive panic sets in, and we might even lose some perspective for a while. Those surrounding a cancer experience can often spend quite some time thinking of ways to make cancer seem less frightening and more under control, just to gain a sense of peace again. This can have us compacting cancer down into a cliché, or else scrambling to find a way to attach some kind of deeper meaning to it. In validating cancer as an experience there to teach us something, it can seem less frightening and arbitrary.

There's nothing wrong with this.

However, as cancer sojourners we need to be mindful we don't simply absorb or accept others projections and conclusions about what our having cancer may "mean", or what lessons we're supposed to draw from it. We also have to be careful not to apply pressure on ourselves to "have it all worked out", or feel obliged to explain to others what deep meaning our having cancer holds, particularly if we don't feel we understand it ourselves, or even want to see cancer that way.

It's perfectly okay to see cancer as a waste of time, totally unfair, and utterly pointless. That's your prerogative.

When you have cancer, people often like to say things such as "The Universe/God is trying to teach you something by giving you cancer. There's a lesson in this for you". And sometimes, the appropriate response to these kinds of remarks is "Really? Then The Universe/God is an asshole."

Sometimes, people like to let you know exactly what lesson they believe your cancer experience has for them, regardless of what your thoughts on the subject are, or what your actual experience may be. After I went into remission I was asked often to speak to groups and at functions about my having cancer. At first I said yes to every invitation - I really wanted to inspire others. But after a few engagements, I became more wary. I realized many folks didn't actually want me to tell the truth about my cancer story - they wanted me to tell the story they wanted to hear about cancer. You see, despite the fact I survived cancer physically, I was significantly traumatized by a delayed diagnosis, and six months of aggressive treatment. I entered remission with a shiny new anxiety disorder. My husband was diagnosed with depression, and was prescribed anti-depressants. I was most definitely not a better person because of cancer, and I found there were people who most definitely did not like to hear about that, not one little bit. After a while, I stopped accepting invitations to speak at events if I suspected they were going to practically hand me a script with what I was supposed to say to make them feel better about my having cancer. I simply didn't feel that way, and I didn't want to lie about it. I wanted to explain how many people were not "all better" once their cancer treatment ended, and how many people who had cancer were tired of being told to 'be positive" all the time But nobody wanted to hear that message.

We can learn a lot from the bad things that happen to us, but only if we want to, and only if there's something to be learned. Sometimes the shit is just the shit, and there's no point, or any higher meaning. Sometimes it's just terrible, ugly and sad, and all we can do is simply allow ourselves to go with it. At times we can extrapolate purpose from our trials, and that is often wonderful, but it isn't ever compulsory.

We all get to choose our own cancer adventure, and it may well be cancer turns out to be the greatest lesson we've ever learned in life. But in releasing our expectations of what cancer must mean, must teach us and must look like, we also release ourselves into our own unique capacity to define cancer in the way which suits us best, instead of allowing cancer to always define who and what we are.

We are always, always better and greater than cancer. And nobody likes being dictated to by something they consider lesser than themselves.

Screw you cancer – you can't tell me what to do.

I'd like to gently suggest you can let go of the script which prescribes how you're supposed to think and act as someone with cancer, and also give you permission not to feel obliged to interpret your cancer journey for others. Let them make of it what they will. You get to choose your own cancer adventure, and do this journey any way you please - noble or cowardly, heroic or needy, changed or unchanged. So much of what happens when you have cancer is out of your control – it's okay for you to take some of that control back again.

This I know - cancer doesn't always have a moral or a point at the end of it. Sometimes it's just a big, fat, waste of time, and that's perfectly okay. Let yourself off the hook, and give yourself a small break. You, and the folks around you will need it now more than ever.

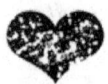

Chapter 3
You Can Change One Thing Today

When cancer comes it can have us feeling disempowered and helpless. Where before we felt we had some control over our life, cancer can have us thinking we have no control at all, and as if any control we thought we had was a lie. But cancer is the liar. Even when something like cancer intervenes we always have choices available to us.

As someone with cancer, we may find ourselves in a position where we need to give power over our body to someone else, but we can still choose to nourish and to nurture ourselves - body, mind and soul. We always retain some choice over what or whom we allow to come close to us right now, and what or whom we'd like to keep at a distance. We can choose not to accept the premise cancer is stronger or greater than we are, and we can also choose to let some things go and hold other things closer. Whilst some choices may be taken away in the wake of a cancer diagnosis, changing our focus can help us recognize areas where we still have control. It's a great feeling knowing whatever happens, you're still in the drivers seat.

Whilst we might feel submitting to the inner work cancer sometimes seems to require of us to be a kind of "giving in", it could well be the issues we're facing would've come up anyway, even if we never had cancer. Illness is often a catalyst for change in areas of our lives which are already problematic, but which we've been able to avoid until now.

Part of surviving is about learning how to keep yourself behind the wheel of your life as you journey through cancer, whilst still accepting the help and support you'll need from others. This can be challenging, particularly if you've been largely independent, or are someone accustomed to leading or caring for others.

Accepting change, help and rest isn't "giving in to cancer" - it's part of helping keep yourself strong. Despite how scared you may feel at the moment, especially if you have more time on your hands than you're used to, don't be afraid to look inwards at your thoughts, feelings and emotions. I'll tell you a secret - cancer won't be found in those deep, inner places. Remember, your body is just one part of you, and there are places - parts of your mind, spirit and soul - cancer cannot touch. In fact, those places may just be about to come into their own. Don't fear the work. You are stronger, braver and kinder than you probably realize, or have been led to believe.

The changes cancer brings can seem overwhelming and catastrophic, particularly at first. Experiencing cancer may seem to take more resources – internal and external - than we think we have to throw at it. But you can do this. Just take one step at a time.

If you are willing, you can change one thing today - one thing which could make all the difference to you in your life, and to others. One small decision could turn this thing right on its head. Exchange one choice you suspect compromises you, for another one bringing you closer to where you want to be. Recovered. Strong. In control. Peaceful. Healthy. Whole. If you don't make yourself a priority, you can't expect others to. Taking the best possible care of yourself is not selfishness. You need you now more than ever before.

Don't look "out there" for the difference - look to yourself. It's not them, or that, or those, or there. It's you. It's in your head, in your heart, in your hands - that's where your future healing and wholeness is, whatever the outcome of the cancer.

Look to your creativity and to your imagination, and not to your past or your history, for the answer to the question "What one change can I make today which will create a difference in this situation for me?"

Today, decide you'll spend a moment to recognize you are the small difference needed in this situation. Don't wait for circumstances or for others to change. Cancer is not in control. You are. Cancer only knows how to do one thing - but you are capable of way, way more.

You can't change the world right now. But you can change one thing today.

Chapter 4

Cancer Never Wins.

There is more than one way for cancer to kill you. Resist cancer physically by all means, but also resist allowing it to convince you it's better or stronger than you. It's not. Ever. Even if you die, cancer is never your better, not even your equal. There is more to you than just the parts cancer can reach.

Cancer never wins.

When somebody dies of cancer, we say, "They lost their battle with cancer", as if between the two of them, cancer was the better, the stronger and the smarter.

But you think about it.

If I die from cancer, cancer dies too.

And if I survive, cancer lost its battle with *me*.

Remember this - **CANCER NEVER, EVER WINS.**

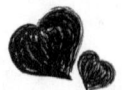

Chapter 5
My Name Is Not Cancer

Before I was diagnosed with stage 3B Non-Hodgkin's Lymphoma in July 2003, my life was pretty darn great. My husband Ben and I and our four children lived in big house in a gorgeous seaside town, where I ran a gorgeous furniture and home wares store. Our children attended the local Christian school, and we were members of a tight-knit community church.

Then one day, after several months of feeling unwell but being fobbed off by my doctor as simply "working too hard", everything changed. I was at work teaching a patchwork class when I began to feel like someone was throttling me in slow, silent increments. Swallowing was like trying to digest a dry sock. My chest rattled when I breathed. Slowly, my consciousness began to slip away. I knew I needed help.

I called Ben, who took me to the nearest hospital. A concerned-looking doctor sent me for an x-ray. After seven months of being dismissed as merely a middle-aged woman with a mild case of gout and a major case of peri-menopausal hysteria, within an hour of being at the hospital they found a tumor the size of a saucer in my chest.

"We're going to need a bigger hospital." said the doctor.

I was in shock, and that was to be expected. But what was not as expected was how quickly I went from being who I was before they found the cancer to something else entirely. People began to see me and treat me differently, immediately.

The doctor at the first hospital who initially greeted me with concern and curiosity, now backed away with a look resembling abject terror on his face.

The friend who came to visit me in hospital, whom we'd shared a glass of wine with just the week before, stood with his hands in his pockets and a look of rank suspicion on his face. "You don't look like someone who has cancer." he said.

Being called "darling", "love", "pet" and "sweetie" even though I was a grown woman with darlings, loves, pets and sweeties of my own. Was I not still an adult?

Being told what a hero I was, when I hadn't really done anything except exactly what everyone in charge told me to do - nothing except lie there and take whatever they did to me. I hadn't been brave. I was scared, confused, angry, often cried like a big sook, told people to go the hell away, and even said I didn't want any more treatment, even if it meant dying of cancer. Why did everyone keep calling me "brave'?

And the worst - being referring to as "the diffused B-cell Non-Hodgkin's Lymphoma". Why did everyone now call me by the same name as the thing I hated, the thing I never asked to get, the thing I was trying so hard to get rid of?

It seemed to me as though everything I was and had achieved before cancer didn't matter any more. I wasn't a grown woman, a mum, a wife or businessperson, and we were no longer just a family of six - we were now, in others eyes, a tragedy in waiting. I was a character in a story, an anecdote people told each other, a cancer victim or a cancer hero.

When you're diagnosed with cancer, it can feel like your identity changes. People often treat and speak to you differently, which can be frustrating, annoying and downright upsetting. People also view you through the lens of their own beliefs and experience of cancer, and if those beliefs and experiences are negative, it can feel as if you're walking around with "CANCER" written in black marker across your forehead.

People avoid looking you in the eye, and when they do, it can seem as if in their minds you already died.

The good news is we don't have to be either the "cancer victim" or "cancer hero" others want us to be. We can teach people how we'd like them to treat us.

If I could go back in time to when I had cancer and tell myself one thing, it would be this:

"Jo - You get to choose how you behave, what you're called, and where cancer sits in the bigger picture of your life. Cancer is something that happened to you - but you are not the cancer."

If someone calls you brave, and you don't feel brave, say so. Describe instead how you do feel.

If someone uses a diminutive to address you such as "sweetheart" just because you have cancer, and this makes you uncomfortable, it's okay to kindly express this.

If someone insists on dropping by at an inopportune time, or wants to visit and you feel uncomfortable about it, politely decline. It's all right to insist on privacy even though you're sick, to say "thank you, but not right now." and close the door.

And perhaps most importantly, find someone you can talk to about how you're really feeling. This may be an empathic friend, cancer coach, social worker, health professional, counselor, psychologist or family doctor.

Let folks gently know whilst cancer is something you're experiencing right now, it hasn't become your new identity. Cancer is happening to your body, but you're still "in there" behind those eyes.

Your name is not and never will be "cancer".

Chapter 6

Letting Others Be Part Of Your Story When You Have Cancer

It can be challenging including others in your cancer experience.

When things are at their worst, we want to protect the people we love from the anxiety and confusion we're feeling. We smile when we feel like crying. We hide behind a locked door, telling folks it's "not a good day". We stay in when we could go out. We change the subject, force a laugh, put on a brave face as they walk in the room - and then take it off again when they go, collapsing from the exhaustion of trying to be one of those who "never complains".

And then there are the times when we just want to punch people in the head for being so nice.

Sometimes, being a cancer "hero" is just bloody hard work.

Nobody wants to be a cancer whiner. We don't even want to hear about it any more, so why would anyone else? Cancer isn't very exciting, not nearly as exciting and interesting as others seem to think. Can't we just change the subject?

"Can I come around and see you?" Can you come around and look at me, you mean. Sure! Bring your friends! You can all go out to lunch afterwards and have something interesting to talk about! OR NOT.

Yep, it's challenging, knowing how to include others in a cancer experience.

There are not many things worse than feeling patronized, placated and pussyfooted around. But as someone with a scary disease, allowing others to come around you and give their offerings to you in the ways they know how is really important for them. It lets them know they have power against cancer too, because they are frightened and feel inadequate and intimidated, just like you. Allowing others near you gives meaning and purpose to them in the cancer, at a time when they may be feeling completely useless and powerless.

They'll ask you later, "do you remember when you were sick, when I....", and you may not even remember what they did and when they did it, but they will. And that matters.

Let go, and let others, even if it's only sometimes. There ain't no medals for doing this solo, you know.

Chapter 7

When 'Support' Means Something Different For Everybody

Last night, I was watching a program about U.S. Marine aircraft carriers commissioned to patrol the ocean around the Middle East in 2005, just a few years after the fall of the World Trade Centre in New York. At one point, a crewmember discussed the general sense of frustration felt at the lack of action or engagement required since they'd been sent there. They were literally all fired up and ready to do...something. Anything - but not *nothing*. Crew who'd known someone personally affected by the events of September 11 wrote a name on each of the bombs which lay waiting in the ships hold. The entire mission was imbued with tension and meaning, each crewmember highly trained, motivated and passionate in their own way. When asked what the orders from above were, one crewmember replied with obvious frustration, "Support. At this time, we're just providing support." From their frustrated demeanor, I could tell the crew of the carrier felt "support" was a relatively benign mission considering what they were capable of, and arrived prepared for. However, my feeling was the civilians living their lives within missile reach of the ship probably viewed the ship, the crew, and the "support" they were there to provide in a completely different way.

When we have cancer, folks around us will often rally with their own unique kinds of "support", but exactly what that entails and how it looks and feels can be a matter of perspective. To the aircraft carrier crew, considering their training, motivation and equipment, providing "support" was a polite way of saying "we're really doing nothing". However the exact same "support", even though it looked like doing nothing, probably felt very different to someone quite else close to the situation.

Sometimes as person with cancer, the support others are capable of and ready to provide isn't the kind we actually want, need or expect. They may turn up with their "aircraft carrier" prepared for an all-out war on cancer, when what we really need is a rowboat, cut lunch and a half-hour of peace and quiet. They may arrive with their comprehensive preparations for battle and even a cancer-fighting bomb with our name on it, when all we really wanted was for someone to listen to us talk about our day without once mentioning the "C" word. They may be equipped to mop our brow, deal with our various nasty ablutions and talk incessantly positive, when what were hoping for was someone to bring us a bottle of wine and laugh with us while we drink it. Sometimes, there's a definite mismatch between how we interpret "support" and how the people around us do, and it may well be what we really want from them doesn't feel like "support" to them at all.

And sometimes, folks will actually avoid us completely because they think supporting a person with cancer requires a fully armed, fully equipped aircraft carrier, and they think their little rowboat is completely inadequate.

Clearly, this can cause all kinds of problems.

People come to cancer with all kinds of fears, expectations, assumptions and ideas. They also come with their genuine good intentions, which often fight for space with the fears and assumptions. As a person with cancer, it's vital for us to be mindful of how the people around us may be feeling not just about our having cancer, but about their own role in our journey. The kinds of "doing" folks who like to see results and enjoy being busy may feel inadequate and frustrated by the situation if they don't find ways to channel their energy. Like the crew of the aircraft carrier, they might assume low-key or passive "support" is a polite way of saying "you're pretty much useless here". Conversely, folks who think cancer happening to you is the biggest, most awful thing that's ever happened to anyone ever might assume they are vastly under-equipped to play a part. They may see "support" as too big an ask, and they might just take their little old rowboat right home and quietly stow it out back in shame and disgust with themselves.

What can we do? It's tricky. People's feelings are often so raw around the subject of cancer; many things are said and unsaid almost subconsciously. But being aware of how others perceive their own capacity to deal with our having cancer is a start. Often, once we broach the uncomfortable silences surrounding cancer and begin to talk about what's really going on, the solutions often become much clearer. Trust in your relationship and what it was like before cancer came, and also what will remain once it's gone, whatever the outcome. This I know - one way or another, with all of us willing and able to pull together to do the work cancer requires of us, everything is going to be okay.

Chapter 8

Finding Out The Deep Meaning Behind Your Having Cancer

I don't remember a whole lot of what I was thinking and how I felt when I had cancer and treatment, because I think I've blotted much of it out. However, there are some thoughts and emotions I do remember having which I now find a little baffling.

It wasn't the being sick part. Pain, long periods in treatment, even death didn't trouble me as much as others probably assumed. When I was diagnosed, I actually felt elated, some might say smug, because I'd been misdiagnosed for months when I knew something was terribly wrong. But having what you'd be forgiven for thinking is the scariest disease in the whole world didn't frighten me as nearly as much as worrying about what on earth I was supposed to be doing as a person with cancer.

What was the higher purpose for me having cancer? What was the special mission I was supposed to be on? Was I doing it right? What if I missed the point? What if my having cancer turned out to be a waste of time?

So obsessed was I with the idea my having cancer was a kind of spiritual quest I'd been sent on, I imagined I was morally obliged to share Jesus with all the other patients in the cancer ward. And when I couldn't do it (because it was, of course, highly inappropriate) I tortured myself with self-shaming until I became even sicker than I already was. As far as I was concerned, if cancer didn't have a higher purpose or meaning for me, and if I didn't have a special job to do while I had it, my cancer experience cancer was totally meaningless.

This thought was simply more than I could bear.

As the months went by, I learned to relax a little. Not because I completely let go of the idea I needed a special job in Cancer World for it to be validated as a meaningful experience in my life, but because I came to see me needing some kind of a special, unique and very energy consuming job while I had cancer would probably be doing a whole bunch of very nice people out of theirs.

I learned I simply had to stop thinking I had a special job to do, and start realizing as a very sick person, I was someone else's special job to do. There were people in my life that raced off to their jobs each day burning with a passion to help people with cancer, just like me. There were people in my world that trained for years to learn how to do the exact things that needed to be done to me to help me get rid of cancer. There were people praying for me, some of them whom I hadn't even met, folks who cried real tears and begged God to intervene as they imagined my kids growing up without their mum. All these folks in my world had a special job to do. My special job for now was to be a sick person who needed these others to help me. Not to help, save and rescue everyone else, but to be helped, saved and rescued.

You may feel your having cancer has no purpose for you in the bigger picture of your life. And it may indeed turn out to be completely pointless and an utter waste of your time and energy. But your having cancer may well turn out to match up exactly with someone else's reason for living. Something to think about.

Chapter 9

Some Negative Thoughts About Positive Thinking

Hey, yo! Person wit cancer! I'm mo make a deal wit ya.

I'll give you one dollar for every time someone says to you "Hey, you just need to think positive!"

Then you and I gonna take a long, expensive cruise to the Bahamas. Deal?

Because we could, couldn't we? How many times have you heard that already?

And how close are you to punching the next person who says you have to think positive right in the head?

I'm joking. About the cruise, and the punch in the head anyway. I'm definitely not joking about the number of times a person with cancer is told - and *told,* as in instructed, as in "you have no choice if you want to help yourself be cured of cancer you must do this" - to think positive. They probably heard about some study proving the effects of positive thinking on cancer. That's okay - most people who insist those with cancer only think happy thoughts speak from this assumption.

It's easy for people who don't have cancer to tell those who do to only think and talk positive. And I mean it - it's very easy for them to say it. I think expecting a person with cancer to only think in a positive way is like asking a hungry person to never ask for something to eat.

As in *cruel and impossible*.

For most people experiencing cancer, the disease and its impacts can very well be the worst thing which ever happened to them. And frankly, telling someone who's experiencing something very, very bad they shouldn't talk about it or else they risk making it worse frankly, isn't very - well - positive.

For someone who has cancer to be unable to speak in a fashion perhaps deemed by others to be "negative" can only really have benefit for the people around them who don't have cancer, because it certainly isn't going to be any good for the one who does. When the person with cancer never talks about the scary parts and is never honest about their fear of pain or death, the only good thing which results is the people around the person with cancer don't have to be inconvenienced with an awkward conversation, deal with their own fear of cancer, or ever confront some of the pressing issues which often need to be faced when someone they love is dying. Like resolution, or forgiveness, or sadness, or loss. No, if we as a person with cancer continue to talk upbeat and deny cancer has the capacity to kill us or destroy anything we value, all of us can keep on living as if everything is just fine.

Except that it isn't just fine. *Somebody has cancer, people.*

The premise regarding positive thinking and cancer has been the subject of various scientific studies, and there are several conclusions available to support both sides of the argument. I can find a couple right now via a reliable internet search engine to prove my position - which is positive thinking has little bearing on cancer outcomes. This is what I think because this is what I've seen.

I've seen people who didn't think positively all the time survive cancer, and I've seen people who did think positively die from it. That's all the evidence I need.

Besides, it's impossible, and unhealthy. You just can't think positively all the time, and nor would you want to.

And what do we even mean when we say "positive"? What does talking negatively about cancer even mean? Does it mean saying things like "I'm worried the treatment won't work." or "I'm afraid of dying"? These are the kind of comments likely to make our loved ones catch their breath in their throat. Do we really believe it could become a self-fulfilling prophecy? Or could it be because these kinds of statements cause us to have feelings and think things we're not ready to confront? Could it be we want a person with cancer to only say and think positive things because we feel inadequate to deal with any negative things? Could it be because we unconsciously want to pretend cancer isn't really happening?

I think this is closer to the truth than we might care to admit.

Besides, do we really think cancer is even listening to the things we say?

One thing I know about cancer - it's about as smart as a pound of wet liver. It's not listening to a dang thing you say. It's just mindlessly doing what cancer does best - multiplying itself, over and over. If thinking positive and happy thoughts were enough to stop cancer doing that, then none of us would ever get cancer in the first place.

When it comes to cancer, the "positive thinking all the time" line of reasoning doesn't really help. Everyone needs to be able to tell the truth about what's happening to them, and express all their thoughts and emotions without criticism. Further, judging our thoughts as "good" or "bad" can cause us to feel we're responsible not just for getting better, but for getting sick in the first place, and also responsible for all the problems being sick caused for us and for others.

Thinking positive may make others feel more relaxed around us, but those negative fears and emotions rarely just disappear. They need to be acknowledged, shepherded, and loved into their place before they become panic or anxiety, because these can cause us to make choices we might not normally make.

Appropriate support and care involves you as a person with cancer being allowed to express your experience and yourself without feeling you'll make cancer worse somehow, or feeling you're responsible for causing it in the first place through something you couldn't help like "negative thoughts". Feeling you did this to yourself will have the effect of undermining your trust in yourself to make good judgments and decisions. It will make you doubt yourself, which is the last thing you need right now. You can absolutely be trusted to make good judgments, and your negative thoughts do not mean you're weak or "bad".

Cancer is bad. You are not.

You are a strong, beautiful and amazing person experiencing something pretty awful right now. And sometimes you're going to need to say out loud, "You know what? This is fucking awful." I suggest you find someone to have this conversation with who isn't threatened or frightened by these kinds of statements, someone who will help you laugh at how stupid cancer really is in the light of fabulous, wonderful you.

And if you've been the kind of person in the past accustomed to saying "Hey, just think positive!" to someone with cancer, perhaps now is a great time for you to instead become the kind of person I just described. Someone who allows their scared, emotional friend to express themselves fully, someone who isn't frightened by conversations about cancer or dying, someone who can help their friend see how truly incredible they are, and who can help them heal, and trust themselves again.

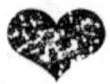

Chapter 10
Telling Yourself The Truth

"The truth will set you free" John 8:32

If there is one thing a person with cancer becomes familiar with, it's fear.

And fear is an asshole.

Also, fear likes hostages.

Anxiety and panic is your imagination held hostage by fear. Once fear gets a hold of your imagination, it'll tie it up and make it watch scary movies.

We won't be able to help but hear our imagination screaming back there in the dark. We'll creep over to see what's going on and, peeking around the corner, we'll see the scary movies playing and realize with horror, "Oh, God, that's me up there!"

The scary movies fear plays to our imagination are all about us and cancer. And because we like and trust our imagination so much, and because it's clearly captive to the fear, we accept those things in the scary movies as true, and real, and actually going to happen to us.

I'm going to die. I need to plan my funeral. They're going to cut me open. No point buying new shoes. I won't see my kids grow up. It's all through me, I just know it. Mum won't cope. I'm not strong. I'm not strong enough. I'm not strong at all. I'm really, really going to die.

I've heard it called catastrophizing - great word.

Catastrophizing is your own fear taking out an insurance policy against you, pretty much. It really is a total asshole.

This is how we end up with panic attacks. Whilst we're busy using all our resources to stay peaceful and calm on the outside, using all the strategies which always worked for us before whenever things were scary or unpredictable before such as toughing it out, sarcasm or plain old denial, our subconscious launches a subversive break-out trying to get us to listen to asshole fear. And when your subconscious starts breaking out, you'll feel it.

Listen to me! Can't you see what's happening? We're being killed with scary thoughts! I will make your heart speed up and trick you into thinking you're having a heart attack! I'll play movies of death and pain in your head until you listen, dammit!

A panic attack is your subconscious trying to keep you alive by making you think you're about to die.

Fight or flight. And away you go.

Now, as a person given to anxiety attacks, I'm not going to offer you any trite cures or remedies for fear, panic or anxiety, because that would be patronizing. What I am going to do is tell you the truth.

Truth is fuel for the creative imagination, which, by the way, you need to go and rescue from fear, right now.

Oh yes, you can. Fear is afraid of the truth. Just take the truth with you, and you'll be fine.

Telling yourself the truth isn't the same thing as positive thinking. Telling yourself the truth means acknowledging fears and concerns without judging them as good or bad, and treating all your emotions with insight, kindness and compassion.

Truth-telling is you punching fear in the head. Your imagination is tied up in the dark, remember? You need to go get that imagination back.

You're going need imagination to help you engineer your hope.

Now, hope engineering is about learning to live from your imagination (with all its powers now used for good and not evil, because you rescued it from asshole fear, remember) and from not your memory, your history or any of those nasty old scary movies about things that haven't even happened yet, and probably never will. Remember - fear can only steal back your imagination if it finds it lying around not being used. Your mission, should you choose to accept it, is to get busy using that fabulous imagination to see a future for you and the people you love based on the truth, and not on any dumb old movies.

What is the truth?

Here are few truths I happen to have handy, just to get you started.

You're doing great, you know.

You're not to blame for all of this.

You're amazing. Even without all your guns blazing, you really are amazing.

You're beloved, and lovely, and loveable.

You're forgiven. Yes, you are.

You can forgive. It's in you.

You're not too much. You never were.

You're significant. Your thoughts, dreams and ideas are significant. What matters to you really does matter in the real world.

You're wise. You know what to do. You can trust yourself.

You didn't let anyone down.

This isn't a punishment.

It's not too late. It's never too late.

It may never happen.

There's no right or wrong way to do this. Your intuition is good. Use it.

There are places in this world cancer cannot reach, and many of those are in you.

Sometimes you have to be your own hero.

Letting go isn't a weakness, and dying isn't a failure.

I believe in you.

Try these truths on for size, and see if any of them open you up inside. Find the ones that do, and feed them to your imagination. There you go - li'l baby bit of hope is being born, right now.

Now you try it.

Chapter 11
You're Okay

A few days after I was diagnosed, we gathered our four kids around the hospital bed and tried to explain that mum had cancer, as best as you can explain to a 15 year old, 11 year old, 9 year old and 3 year old. As our youngest rolled with glee across the blanket, we solemnly explained that mum was very sick, but we were going to do everything we could to get me well again. We also explained how it might be I didn't get better, or get to come home again, but we weren't going to think about that right now. We would just do today, and we'd just do today, every day. And no matter what happened - no matter what happened - everything was going to be okay.

Years later, I asked my eldest about what he was thinking around that time. "I knew whatever happened, no matter how afraid I was, even if you died, everything was going to be okay."

Was our response to my diagnosis normal? Was their reaction normal? Normal? Mum having cancer and possibly going to die? Never. There was nothing normal about our children being put through that.

But were they okay?

We told them whatever happened, whatever they felt, wanted to do, needed to express, pulled closer to or let go of, it was okay.

Even if I never came home again, they were going to be okay.

The situation was not normal, and thinking about whether it was normal, right or fair wasn't going to help any of us. Instead we told our kids they would be afraid and there was nothing wrong with that. We also told them no matter what happened to mum we would find a way to help them feel safe again.

They would feel safe again.

They were okay.

Here are some of the things I am asked most frequently by people who have cancer, or had cancer -

"I don't think I can ever go back to the way things were before cancer. Is this normal?"

"It's difficult for me to trust my body now, after all, I feel it let me down. Is this normal?"

"My friends seem to be over my having cancer, and I know I'm not. Is this normal?"

"I sometimes wake up in the night so anxious and scared I can't breathe. I feel like I'm going to die. Is this normal?"

"My friends tell me I've changed. I'm just not interested in doing the things we used to enjoy. Is this normal?"

"I just want to forget cancer ever happened. Is this normal?"

"I'm a wreck. Is this normal?"

"I'm perfectly okay. Is this normal?"

And I say "Normal? Probably not. But is it okay? Absolutely."

When it comes to cancer, and the other terrible things that can happen to us, there is no such thing as "normal", old, new, or otherwise. But there is such a thing as "okay".

There is no use telling you your feelings are abnormal or wrong and you need to correct them. There is no benefit to you in me trying to make you into the same person you were before cancer. There is no "getting back to normal." How will you know if you ever get there?

But it's completely different when we talk about being okay. When I say, "you're okay", what I mean is I'm not judging the way you live your life, your thoughts and emotions or your choices as good or bad. They are what they are. They're all yours, and they're all valid.

What you're feeling is okay. What you want and don't want are also okay. What you feel you can't do is okay, and what you want to do is also okay. There will be things you do now you regret later, and things you don't do you'll regret, but it's all okay. It really is. Forget about normal. What's normal anyway? If you abide by statistics, then something happening to every second person in the general population - like cancer - could be said to be "normal."

Is cancer normal?

Did it feel anything like what normal is supposed to feel like to you?

Let's just forget the concept of normal, and let's go for okay instead, okay?

Is cancer okay? Is having cancer okay? Absolutely not.

Are you okay? Yes, you are. Is everything you think and feel because of cancer okay? Sure is. Will everything be okay, regardless of what happens, or whether everything goes back to how it was before?

I believe so.

When it comes down to it, you're probably not normal.

But you're okay.

Chapter 12
Not My Time

Today, a friend asked me:

"Name something you did today with all your heart."

It was an easy question to answer.

Today, I wrote some words about another day a few years ago - the day I decided I wanted to be fully alive for the rest of my life.

I was about halfway through my radiotherapy treatment, and the most ill I've ever been. Three months of chemotherapy, a stem cell harvest, blood transfusion, six weeks away from my family and a very nasty case of shingles on top of everything had pulled me down further than I'd been in my life, physically, emotionally and mentally. I honestly felt like dying was a reasonable, comfortable option, if going on living was going to be anything like that.

I slept - thank God, I slept - and dreamt of swimming. I swam laps and laps, up and down, all the time watching the bottom of the pool, wondering what it would be like to live down there. After swimming laps in my dream for what seemed like hours, I wanted to stop and just rest a while.

At the end of the last lap I didn't tumble turn, instead letting myself just sink into the deep end. I slowly drifted to the bottom, unafraid, happy to be at rest. In my dream, I stopped breathing. I let my arms and legs just hang there. I closed my eyes and started to drift away. *Just what I need - a long, long sleep.*

Suddenly, I'm startled by a sound – a voice - a muffled scream. I feel a boiling in my throat. It's my voice. I'm screaming.

I shake myself awake from the dream. *No, not now. It's not my time. This is not when I get to stop living.* I must keep on being alive, and only I can do it. Keep swimming, keep going. This will not last forever. Keep breathing, keep going. Don't stop now.

I dredge my soul up heaving from the bottom of myself. I know it was close, as close as it gets, but here I am.

I love today, every today, because every today I am here to write about that other day when I had the choice whether to hold out for a day like this. I will never cease to be astonished at how bright and close every day is to me now. I don't have to swim so hard anymore, but the practice has made me lean and strong - strong enough to hold my own, and others' too. Strong enough to bear to remember when death whispered in my ear and made me think that sleeping would be better than waking, sinking better than swimming, dying better than surviving.

Name one thing I did today with all my heart?

I lived.

Chapter 13
Creativity And Cancer

I'm a writer. I've always written. I've written all kinds of stuff - stories, advertising copy, commentary, sermons, songs, you name it. I've never had any trouble writing - oh, except for that time I found I couldn't write, no matter how much I wanted to.

When I had cancer.

So much to write about, and yet, when it came to writing it all down, I was dry as old bones. It was like that part of my brain went into chemical hibernation. I simply couldn't access the part where beautiful, sensible words came from. So I went about it another way. Instead of trying to write lines and verses, I wrote single words, one after the other. It was all I could do, so I did it.

Here's a poem I wrote from that time about the way I felt during chemotherapy -

Dying dreaming drifting

Speaking shouting screaming

Whispering praying wishing

Holding slipping falling

Spinning sliding sleeping

Thinking doing walking

Waking reaching knowing

Growing feeling flowing

Flailing gripping gritting

Bruising bleeding crying

Resting smiling sailing

Blowing breezing waving

Diving deepening drifting

Dreaming drowning

Dying

It was a particularly difficult time.

Despite the fact I struggled to write anything back then, I pore over those scribblings now searching for clues as to my state of mind, my thoughts and my emotions. I wasn't giving much away. I do remember feeling it was somehow wrong to whine and be scared, to admit I wasn't getting any answers to the questions I asked of God. I felt my art should be positive and filled with meaning. I wish I hadn't bothered worrying about that. I wish I'd just let myself pour it all out and permitted myself to go to those depths, to tell the truth about how I was thinking and feeling.

Clearly, I'm making up for it now.

I know how hard it can be to express yourself emotionally and creatively when you're going through something like cancer and treatment. You can feel like everything you write or think is rubbish, literally to be thrown away and forgotten. But everything we think and feel in the midst of experiences like cancer is valid, and significant. I look back on those scraps of writing I made and I see something I rarely saw before in my writing before I had cancer - I see the real me, the me that came through it, the authentic, vulnerable, tough me - the me that once lived on the inside, but lives on the outside now. Treatments like chemo are designed to kill off every newborn cell in your body in the hope of interrupting the growth of cancer cells too - and it can feel like a soul death as well as a cell death at times. It can feel like a spiritual and artistic suffocation. But sometimes all it takes is a little prompting, a little permission, a little puff of fresh air for the smothering pall of death to be blown away and inspiration to come back into your soul again.

Come on back to life, sweetheart. Let's start making things again.

Here are some ways you can wake up your soul and help your body and spirit start to sprout some new growth:

Begin a journal. Resolve not to try and make it pretty or make sense, just tell it like it is.

Have a go at writing poetry. If you find you struggle, try writing just one word at a time, like I did with my poem. You may be surprised how powerful this is.

Try cryptic crosswords, or other kinds of puzzles. Creativity isn't just about art. Creative thinking involves finding new ways of doing things. Teach your brain to seek a different route to a solution by taking it places it's never had to go before. Challenge your mind and it'll reward you by building new synapses and bridging new connections in your brain. Teach yourself to see problems differently and to respond to them in new, creative ways.

Pick up a musical instrument and just play around. Don't go for excellence. Just let each sound the instrument makes vibrate through you. A guitar is great, because you have to hold it against your body. It's like a massage for your cells. Playing even simple music also teaches your brain it's safe for you to have adventures and take risks, and you can trust in your ability to improve your skills and master new things.

Attend a concert or performance. Your body and mind will just love it.

Begin a quilt. Tell others you're stitching and want some beautiful, good quality fabrics to get you started. Find a group in your area and join.

Sing. Sing along to the radio, or your favorite CD. Join an accapella singing group. Again, the vibration of the singing - yours, and others - is great for your cells. It will encourage new cell growth and stimulate endorphins, making you feel better all over.

Paint, draw, and sketch. All you need is paper or canvas and inexpensive paints. If you don't know what you're doing, just put color down and swirl it around. Sign on for a class. Stretch yourself artistically into new mediums, new methods.

Make a collage of inspiring images from magazines or the internet. Create an account on Pinterest and go crazy with it. Spend time every day intentionally looking at images you find evoke in you a sense of hope, wonder, joy and optimism. Conversely, you could find images representing your perception of cancer or the way you're feeling as a way of acknowledging your feelings and mindsets. Find a way to change the way those images look – tear them into pieces and make a mosaic or a mandala from them, for example.

Remember - cancer cannot make anything new. It can only mindlessly replicate itself over and over. But you are an amazing, creative being. You can make something that never existed before just from your imagination, with your hands, with your breath or movement or voice. Make it your intention to bring something into the world today which wasn't here yesterday, something original and new, even if it's simple, small or not made with a great deal of skill. It doesn't matter. We talk about cancer as if it were stronger and more powerful than we are, but cancer can't make anything original or beautiful. Anything you birth into reality through your creativity, no matter how humble or small, is going to be a whole world more awesome than anything cancer can ever do.

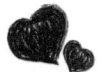

Chapter 14
How To Be An Inspiration

Whenever I go speak to a group or at an event, I never take any new material. I've learned the cleverer or more authoritarian I pretend to be on a subject, the bigger a wanker I appear, and the harder it is to keep on pretending to be wonderful when I get down from the platform. When it comes to my subject of choice, I'm no expert. I don't bring anything new to the conversations I have or the stuff I write about cancer. Its all been said and done before.

The only thing I can bring people they haven't heard before is my story, truthfully told.

The other day, I was having a particularly hard time at my job (I work as a sales assistant in a dress shop). Christmas shoppers can be particularly belligerent. I know why this is - everyone is spending too much money, and feeling the weight of expectation to make Christmas into some kind of joy orgy - but it doesn't make dealing with the cold glares and icy rebuttals from customers any easier to deal with. I was feeling particularly dispirited, when a lady who was trying on a couple of dresses poked her head out from behind the curtain and said to me, "I know you. Didn't you speak at a cancer advocacy conference a few years ago in Sydney?"

"Sure did." I replied.

"I thought it was you! Hey, I just wanted to tell you it was one of the most inspiring things I've ever heard in my life. Honestly."

Tears sprang to my eyes. My self-esteem, which had been stuck like dog poop to the sole of my shoe, wafted back up and seeped back into my heart like steam off honeyed tea.

I thanked her for making my day.

I was thinking about what it means to be inspiring on the way home from speaking at a cancer support group this morning. I'm often introduced as an "inspiring speaker", but a long time ago I stopped thinking there was something special I could be or say to make people be inspired. I didn't set out to be an inspiration, although it can be a little bit addictive having people say you are.

According to my dictionary, "inspire" means "to fill (someone) with the urge or ability to do or feel something". It literally means, "to put the spirit in". We can try to inspire with stunningly innovative information or wild tales of our derring-do. But what happens when someone is inspired has little to do with what we say. It happens because of what we are. We inspire others whenever we truly reach someone's spirit with our spirit.

I've come to the conclusion people will not be inspired by our specialness, our greatness, our peculiar talent, strength or courage. People will be inspired when their heart has been accessed and they believe they have truly accessed our heart. This is what I know - honesty, authenticity and a willingness to simply tell the truth about ourselves absolutely changes others' lives.

Don't seek greatness, expertise or uniqueness in the hopes it will inspire others. Your knowledge is useless if they don't feel you're accessible. Don't seek to know more on your topic than anyone else, simply seek to grow your capacity to be honest and authentic, and expand your willingness to be vulnerable.

Nobody was ever encouraged by a lie, or a liar.

When people feel they have connected with your true spirit, it will bring them to life in ways both you and they cannot even imagine.

Chapter 15
Your Story Matters

We love stories.

There are many reasons why people love stories. Stories connect us. They inform us. They help us feel like we're okay. They excite us, inspire us. They comfort us, and illuminate the past and the future. They make us feel special. They help us realize we're not alone.

What happened to me happened to them.

That's just like me.

I feel that way.

I want to do that.

That'll be me one day.

I know what that's like.

This is who I am.

This is where I belong.

Stories connect us - to place, to people, to experience, to culture, history and to each other.

Indigenous cultures understand the vitality and importance of story, and not just the individual story - the collective story.

The story of me, and the story of us.

There is an intrinsic power in story we can access and use, but we must overcome any beliefs we hold which dictate telling others about ourselves is something resembling pride, conceit, narcissism, self-centeredness or ego.

Those mediocrity-maintaining, self-preserving habits may have served us well in the playground or the classroom or some other hostile environment, but our story may turn out to be far more powerful than we can imagine.

Your story is important, significant, and infinitely interesting.

People are hurting. We are hurting. We need each-others stories.

Someone needs your story.

Yes, your story matters.

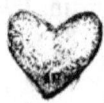

Chapter 16

Your Wonderful, Powerful, Imperfect Story

We live in a success oriented society. On the whole, we highly value perfection, excellence, progress and achievement.

We're encouraged to plan and organize our lives at every juncture and in every respect to best place ourselves for this success we value so highly, as well as for efficiency and effectiveness. "Fail to plan, plan to fail." they say, and we believe it.

Because failing at something is the worst thing that could ever happen, right?

We're compelled to dream our most wonderful life whilst at the same time subjugating it into a rigid, formulaic and logical narrative, as if our whole human experience could be simply lined up and trotted out neatly like chapters in a book.

In fact, whole books, programs and seminars have been designed around the premise we should, and can, "write our life like a story".

But what happens when our story takes an unexpected and very unpleasant turn? What happens when that marvelous plot, good organization, superb administration, meticulous planning and logical order are thwarted by something random and uncontrollable?

Like cancer?

The "worst thing that could ever happen" happens, that's what.

The "f" word.

Failure.

The problem with thinking you can plan your life like a story is the fact nobody in their right mind is ever going to write in any shitty parts if they actually have to live that story.

Would you write cancer, or a car accident or a miscarriage or a divorce for that matter, into your own story? Of course not.

Do people in the real world - not in super-amazing-rainbows-and-unicorns-plan-your-life-like-a-story world - get cancer?

Statistics say one in two folks in the general population do. Are the rest just very well organized?

An awful lot of people who find out they have cancer are walking around feeling as though they've been very poorly organized. In fact, they feel like failures. They think they and their stories are flawed, imperfect and broken. But this isn't true. You see, a story without any expected turns, without risk or tension or threat or failures isn't actually a story.

It's a filing system.

Your life isn't an exam to be passed. It isn't a menu to be perused and chosen from, with only excellent choices available. It isn't the road you're travelling down, the gravel and the tar and the white lines painted down the middle to tell you which side to keep on. Life is the journey you make while you're on that road, with all the turns and the scenery, the stops, starts and yes, the turns, expected and unexpected alike.

You can't plan your life like you write a story. Nobody wants a life with any of the things in it that make a good story interesting or worth something to others. If we had to live the kinds of stories we actually have the stomach to write for ourselves, we'd find ourselves constantly falling asleep at the wheel.

I believe in the power of story. Not "story" the militant life-coaching regime, or "story" the magical-thinking formula for perfection, or "story" the nothing-to-see-here, all-the-bad-parts-written-out movie script. I believe in story, the real thing.

Story. You talking about the stuff that really happens to real people in the real world, regardless of how well organized we are - the stuff which happened to you.

Story. The imperfections and the flaws, the scars and the wounds tenderly revealed and gently touched upon with compassion and acceptance, instead of with judgment, distaste and disdain.

Story. All the things connecting you to others, and they to you, instead of us all set up against one other in a kind of competition for impossible perfection.

Story. Reflecting on the past and dreaming of the future knowing we only have so much control, and there is bittersweetness in the chaos, as well as in the order.

Stories connect us and inform us. They help us feel like we're okay. They excite us, inspire us, comfort us and illuminate the past and the future.

Your story has value simply because it's yours. It doesn't have to be perfect, or need a moral or message to matter, or to be powerful.

Stories let us know we're not alone in our frailties, imperfections and flaws, and even more than we need to feel perfect, successful and less like failures, we need to know we're not alone.

Your story matters, mostly to the other folks out there who feel their stories are flawed, and they are failures, because of cancer.

Tell your story.

Chapter 17
Your Burning, Broken, Beautiful Story

Talking about yourself is hard.

Talking about the worst thing that ever happened to you is even harder.

Talking about yourself, and the worst thing that ever happened to you, which also happens to be the one thing the mere mention of which generally sends people crashing backwards across the room, out the door and halfway down the street is the hardest. I don't care who you are, it just is.

This is why an awful lot of people - probably more than you realize - will never tell anyone they have cancer. Maybe not even when it's happening.

Cancer and treatment can be lonely, difficult and stressful. It's stressful for others around us as well. Often, the reason we don't want to talk about cancer is because it upsets the people who care about us. Even if we managed to cope quite well with the experience, our having cancer may be the worst thing that ever happened to our friends or family, and they may never want to hear about it again.

Not talking about cancer may be our way of assuring folks everything is all right again, and normal life has returned.

Not telling anyone about your having cancer, even when you have it, can have its benefits. But there are times when telling people your story is going to be worth the trouble, if not for you, then for the person you're telling your story to.

There is more than one way for cancer to make us "sick." We can be heartsick. Soul sick. Brainsick. Friend sick. Cancer can hurt us in a plethora of ways, other than the obvious physical ones. I know, because I got all these kinds of sick when I had cancer, and more besides.

When I had these ten kinds of sick because of cancer, I really needed contact with another human being who understood what I was going through. More than I needed to hear the cliché's like "what doesn't kill you makes you stronger!" more than I needed to stay positive or know how much longer I could expect to live beyond my treatment, I really needed someone who would sit with me and tell me I wasn't broken because of my thoughts and feelings – someone who could say "I know", and mean it. It was hard for me to find that kind of help, because many of the folks who'd been where I was had kicked out running and never looked back. Many folks who'd been through cancer didn't want to go back into the "cancer world", because getting better for them meant leaving it behind. But I knew I needed someone who didn't just read about the ten kinds of sick I had in a book. I needed someone who truly understood, who spoke the language and recognized the landscape. I needed someone who'd been there.

Now, even though I've been through cancer and treatment, I can't know exactly what you've been through. But I do know this. At some stage, someone is going to ask you about it. Someone is going to want to know what you did when you had cancer and how you did it, and it won't just be a morbid fascination. It'll be because this one feels as though they've just returned from a foreign land, and they just heard you speak a few words of the language. It'll be because they're frightened and feel desperately alone, and all the folks they love look so terrified and helpless whenever they try to talk to them about how they feel. It will be because you represent something they desperately want to believe exists.

The future.

You'll become a symbol of hope.

And one day, somebody's eyes will swing around to meet yours, and you'll see in those eyes the familiar fear you faced before, and you'll want to run away, but your heart will remember that loneliness and terror and compassion will overcome you. And someone will ask you if you'd mind having your picture taken for the local paper, because they'd like to run a story about cancer to raise awareness or raise money. Count on it. And one day, you'll find out that people with cancer in your town can no longer have access to a treatment you were given because someone changed the rules, or someone decided to pull funding, and you'll become hot with anger and indignation about it, and you'll want to go out and give someone a piece of your mind. And you'll think about how talking about yourself is hard, and talking about the worst thing which ever happened to you is harder, and talking about yourself and cancer in the same sentence may well be the hardest thing you could ever do. But then you'll realize you probably already did the hardest thing you'll ever do. And you'll know then in that moment, telling your story is just what you need to do.

You survived, you're surviving, and you are a survivor. You did and are doing something very, very hard. People need help, and they also need hope. You don't learn about how to give people hope out of a book, in a class or from an expert. You learn to give others hope by very almost losing it, and then getting it back again.

You can give people hope. Your story matters. Tell your story.

Chapter 18

Cancer Winners and Losers, Fighters and Survivors

One of the hardest things about surviving cancer is realizing you can't actually take much credit for it.

I know this flies directly in the face of the "cancer hero" myth, but it's true. Let's just be honest - when it comes to cancer there are only two possible outcomes, and cancer survivors by default end up with the only outcome which ever requires an explanation.

And survivors are asked for the explanation for how we survived cancer whether we have one or not.

And if we don't have one, someone else is sure to provide us with one they just happen to have handy. Because it's assumed we "won our fight against cancer" just because we're still alive and didn't die. And the ones who aren't here to provide an explanation are said to have "lost their battle". Because folks generally assume we who get well again are the winners, and the ones who didn't are -

losers?

Despite the cliché, it just doesn't work that way.

We all go in determined to fight cancer. But not all the fighters survive. And not everyone who starts out fighting keeps on fighting, and not all the ones who stop fighting die when they do. Not everyone who gets well again did so because they fought harder than someone who died. Some give up fighting, and live to tell about it. Some fight and fight and fight, and go down fighting, and don't get up again. And just as many die fighting as live having given up fighting.

Fighting cancer, as it turns out, doesn't really make a lot of difference to the outcomes. You still only get one of the two regardless of how much fighting you do, and how hard you do it. Despite this, we still we talk about people who survived cancer as having done something clever or praiseworthy, and people who die from cancer as having given in, been defeated, or just plain old lost their battle with cancer.

So as a survivor, people ask me a lot "So, what did you *do*?"

They want to know what I did to survive cancer, because I'm still alive, so clearly whatever I did worked. Naturally, everyone wants a solution to cancer that works.

Truth is, I don't take any credit for getting physically well again. I did what I was told. I didn't fight cancer, because I didn't understand what fighting cancer actually meant, when all I did was lay around and do what others told me and allowed people to do things to me they said would get rid of cancer. I do, however, consider myself a cancer survivor.

Surviving cancer for me wasn't about not dying, although I certainly didn't want to die. Surviving was about not letting cancer kill me in all the other ways it had the potential to, other ways with not much to do with whether I stayed in this world or left it. I figured when it came to actually dying, I'd just cross that bridge when I came to it.

Surviving is something completely different from not dying of cancer.

Surviving for me means having the courage to change the way I was living my life, because I believed cancer came about as a result of choices I'd made I had no business choosing, and paths I'd walked down I had no business walking down. Nothing to do with not dying.

Surviving means getting help for my crippling fear and anxiety - the legacy of being misdiagnosed for seven months then thrown into treatment four hundred kilometers away from my home and family less than a week after I was diagnosed. Again, not *not dying*.

Surviving means acknowledging my marriage wasn't going to, and reminding myself I'd been alone and in pain before, and I could damn-well do it again if I had to.

Surviving means watching almost everyone I met while I was sick, and many, many more in the years that followed, fight, and not live while I lived on.

Surviving means being absolutely determined not to allow that which almost killed me define me, or be the most interesting thing to ever happen to me.

Surviving means making sure people don't consider me a winner just because I didn't die of cancer.

Surviving also means making sure people don't talk about all my friends who died from cancer as losers just because they aren't here to talk about all the ways they fought and survived and won.

Be this change, with me, will you?

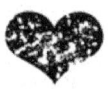

Chapter 19
We Feel It All

When you've had cancer, people assume you're tougher than most, or at the very least, tougher than you were.

"You're amazing. You're so strong. I could never go through what you've been through."

But people do go through it. All kinds of people go through cancer. Strong, weak, ready, or not - everyone diagnosed with it must go through it. We don't have a choice.

Folks who haven't been through cancer can only imagine what kinds of things we actually have to experience. Knowing you have cancer and could die is scary and often painful, for sure. But some of the things they have to do to you to get rid of it are even scarier, and more painful.

This week, I was listening to a twelve year-old cancer coaching client tell me what for him was the scariest parts.

"Hearing I had cancer was scary. But the worst parts were when they gave me a bone marrow biopsy, and when they put in my central line (the tube in his chest through which chemotherapy goes). Mum, they'll knock me out when they take out the central line, won't they?"

I remember my own bone marrow biopsy. "This won't hurt" the technician assured me as she pushed the needle with all her might into my hipbone. I felt a grinding sensation, and it hurt.

I remember after I'd been in remission for twelve months and some of my CT scan results came back with a report contradicting the scans. My oncologist rang to clarify. "I need to know if you made a mistake on this report before I send this woman back to hospital and they stick a foot long needle into her chest to find out if you made a mistake or not." I closed my eyes, nausea and panic chasing each other up my throat. They'd stuck a foot long needle into my chest before, twice. Both times I was fully conscious.

They never told me sometimes I'd feel like the people who were there to fix me were trying to murder me. I now have a letter from my doctor stating if they need to stick a foot-long needle into my chest again, I need to be unconscious when they do it.

We seem tougher, we folks who've had cancer. Perhaps we don't get as scared by roller coasters or as upset when people do stupid things to us as we used to. It looks like strength, but it's more likely to be distraction. We're not frightened by the prospect of hanging upside down strapped into an amusement park ride, because our particular universe now includes the possibility of having foot long needles driven into various parts of our body whilst we're told to hold still by people who claim to be helping us and not actually murdering us. Our particular reality encompasses now the greatest threat to our life coming from inside our own cells, not from being hit by a bus or bitten in half by sharks. What looks like strength is really just an expanded view of the terrible things that can really happen to people, and realizing they can come from places that are very, very close by, and from people you like and trust who will smile and say, "this won't hurt."

With and after cancer, we're still terrified. Sometimes even more terrified than we were before. Terrified by the possibility of things happening most people cannot even conceive of.

"But you could be hit by a bus tomorrow" folks say, trying to allay what they consider to be our irrational fear of the illness recurring. They say this because being afraid of being hit by a bus is, in their mind, an irrational fear. I imagine this fear is a little more rational for someone who has actually been hit by a bus.

It looks like a phobia, but it's not a phobia if it's actually happened, and if there is any realistic probability it could happen again.

And what happens when the bus, the road and the accident are inside your own body?

People often assume because we've had cancer, we're stronger and tougher than we were. The truth is we may be more resilient in some areas, but may actually more scared and much weaker in others. Our confidence in our body, and our ability to simply assume bad things just won't happen to us, may be shaken and never return, but our confidence to ride roller coasters and our resilience in inclement circumstances may be increased.

"My body let me down. It may do again. If it does, scary things will happen to me, and I won't be able to control those. But time is short, and roller coasters are fun."

Our tolerance for crap may be decreased. Our willingness to allow ourselves to be subject to pain, abuse and attack may be diminished. This can look like weakness, and it can look like strength, and it's probably both. It's also self-preservation.

"My marriage is just bloody hard work. It shouldn't be this hard. I'm worth better than this."

Once you've felt pain right through to your marrow, you'll do anything to avoid that kind of pain ever happening again.

We who've had cancer look tough. We seem tough. But trust me - we feel it all.

Chapter 20
Make Cancer Pay

This, my friend, is the day I want you to turn it around.

There are so many things you can't change right now. You're so deep in it - those things you can't control are perhaps all you can think about.

I have cancer. Things will never be the same again.

I know it seems unfair, this heightened sense of what is and really isn't important. But honestly, this is how we're supposed to live. *For now, for today.* But we don't. You're now realizing how short time really is, how little time you have.

Don't lose that. I promise you, keeping that one thing will change your life.

Today, my friend, today we flip this.

You have the following choice before you, and you can make it.

You will make it, whether you mean to or not.

Will cancer be the worst thing that ever happened to you?

Will you give that kind of power to cancer? It is a kind of "giving over" power - making something the worst, the hardest, the toughest or the most destructive. When you speak this way, you give cancer power.

Power, frankly, it doesn't deserve.

Will cancer be the worst thing that ever happened to you? Or will cancer be something else?

Cancer can kill your body. But it cannot kill who you are, what you are.

You have the choice - you can think about what cancer takes away from you, or you can think about what you can take away from cancer.

Cancer comes to rob, steal and destroy. It makes you pay - with your body, with your mind, with your wellbeing and your future.

But today, it changes. Today you make up your mind that from now on - *cancer pays*.

Make it famous. Cancer hates it when you talk about it like it's an everyday thing. Talk about cancer without shame or fear, or even guilt because of anything you might have done to make it come. Cancer doesn't want to be famous - it wants to stay nameless, secretive and mysterious. It needs these so it can infect you and everyone you know with fear, killing you all in a hundred awful ways. Make cancer famous, and take away its safety and anonymity.

Make it smaller. Cancer isn't bigger than you; so don't behave as if it is. Laugh at its expense. You have a greater capacity to get rid of cancer than it has to get rid of you. Even if it takes your body, it becomes extinct. You always win. Make cancer smaller, because it's never your greater, never even your equal.

Make it normal. Yes, normal. One in two folks are diagnosed with cancer - so why are we still acting as if having cancer is rare, unique and unlucky? Something happening to every second person isn't special. The myth of cancer thrives on us continuing to believe it's an anomaly. One in two people means it's less to do with being unlucky, and more to do with being human. The more we behave as if cancer is part of life, the less special and potent it becomes. Make cancer normal, and take away its power.

Make it pay. Use cancer in ways it never counted on. Cancer isn't a weakness - it's a unique skill set. Cancer teaches you stuff you can use to help others beat it, or at the very least, negotiate it. Knowing what the inside of the cancer world looks like opens doors for you, doors you can jimmy open and shepherd others through, doors that one day won't exist because people like you will wrench them off their hinges and throw them away. Get yourself on a platform because of cancer, and use it to tell people not to believe the myths and the lies. Get your photo in the paper, and tell people your own amazing story. Make cancer pay, and suck every damn shred of fame and airtime you can screw out of it to wage a campaign of forced extinction against it.

Today, we turn this thing around. Make up your mind to think less about what cancer can take away from you, and begin to strategize what you can take away from it. Make it into a unique and specialized skill set. Force it out into the light. Make it clear and obvious to anyone who'll listen exactly what cancer has done, and also, what it can never do.

Make cancer smaller. Make cancer normal. Make cancer pay.

Chapter 21
Curing "Burnt Toast" Syndrome

A few months before I found out I had cancer (I was ill for quite some time before I could get someone to listen to me) I presented to my local chemist with some puzzling symptoms, one of which was a terrible pain in the ball of my right foot. The pharmacist behind the counter diagnosed me immediately with gout - an accumulation of uric acid crystals in the joint. Horrified at finding out I had something with such an unglamorous name, I asked him what caused it.

"Burnt Toast Syndrome."

"I beg your pardon?" I imagined I'd contracted a terrible disease caused by too many toxic enzymes in my overcooked breakfast. "What exactly is Burnt Toast Syndrome?"

"Burnt Toast Syndrome" he explained, "is when someone capable and with a lot on their plate takes responsibility for the happiness of everyone else, and always puts themselves last on the list. In other words, I think you always take the "burnt piece of toast" so nobody else around you ever has to feel inconvenienced, disappointed or unhappy. Am I right?"

He was right.

Burnt Toast Syndrome didn't give me cancer. But after I found out I had cancer, it became pretty clear Burnt Toast Syndrome wasn't going to help me get better.

I had to learn it was important for me to take the "freshest piece of toast" more often, and leave the burnt one for someone else, because sometimes others need to learn when to put someone else's wants and needs before theirs. I also needed to make my own happiness and comfort a priority as well as that of my family and friends, and stop seeing personal sacrifice and self-denial as noble, or a sign of my love. Teaching others to respect my health and happiness wasn't wrong, and allowing the people in my life to experience disappointment or inconvenience as I moved myself up my list of personal priorities wasn't selfish or bad.

Having cancer was an opportunity for me to learn to practice self-nurture, because I could hardly expect others to take better care of me than I was prepared to take of myself.

In fact, making martyrs of ourselves may be one of the factors that promote ideal conditions for problems like cancer. If you constantly put yourself at the bottom of the list, you're bound to become sick - if not physically, then perhaps in some other way.

You don't get a different result by continuing to make the exact same choices. Today, it's time to cure yourself of "Burnt Toast Syndrome". Looking after yourself properly and partaking of good food and healthy, fulfilling activity isn't wrong, selfish or bad. Listen to what your body is telling you. Something you've been doing isn't working. Time for a change.

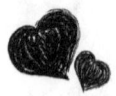

Chapter 22
You're Going To Make It

This isn't going to last forever, my friend.

It came from nowhere, didn't it? It came from inside you, and not from the outside, where scary things are supposed to come from. They're supposed to be under the bed, around the corner, in the closet, in that spooky house across the street, with that car careening down the road. Scary things are supposed to be avoidable - don't look, don't go there, don't follow along with that person or do that stupid thing, and there you go - nothing to be scared of. Scary things aren't supposed to be inside your body. Scary things aren't supposed to be made of you.

How could you not know? How could you not stop it? How can you not make it go away by just avoiding it, or crossing the street or closing the closet? How did this come to have its beginning in you? Tell me, and I'll stop doing it. Tell me, because everyone keeps asking, "So, do you know what caused it?" I know they want to avoid the scary thing too. How can I tell them where it came from? Just how do you explain that?

And then there's what happens when you stop being scared, and you start to get accustomed to the fact you have cancer. There's what happens when you've been all the way through shock and terror and the realization you could die, and out the other side. When your body decides there's no point pushing all that energy into emotions any more, and makes up it's mind that your calories and serotonin would be better used doing other things like keeping you calm, or making healthy cells, or repairing the effects of chemotherapy. And you wonder why you don't get happy or sad anymore, and why you can't stay focused on a movie or an interesting project, and you start to wonder if this what it feels like to start dying.

And then there's what happens when you begin to wonder what on earth is real and right and true any more, and what you can trust and what you can't, and what this means about the way things are in this world, and the kinds of things that can happen to people, even good people. And you think about the future, but you can't see it the way you used to either in your head or your imagination, or wherever it is hope is made. And you wonder, "is this a sign?" Does it mean you won't live to see your graduation, or your wedding, or their graduation or their wedding, because you just don't dream like that any more? And you wonder, is this what *survival* means - living the rest of your life with an erased imagination, with shallow dreams, with hope that only extends in minutes and hours and days, and not in years and lifetimes?

This feels like it's going to last forever, my friend. But it isn't. You're reading this because it doesn't last forever. I've been there - and here I am. The flat, dreamless existence you're dragging yourself through now will one day be a memory. This isn't going to be your life. You're going to make it. You'll make it home. To the graduation and the wedding. To the birth, to the first day of school, to the birthdays and the holidays and the cake and the photos and the laughter. You'll be there.

This isn't going to last forever, my friend. You're going to make it.

Chapter 23
No More Dramas

No more dramas.

No, no more dramas. Who needs them? Life is hard enough, and besides, we just don't have that kind of time.

You have better things to do with your time and energy.

Promise yourself right now - I solemnly vow, *I will no longer create dramas for myself.*

No more dramas to get what you want, and no more to avoid what you don't.

No more dramas to make people think you have something worth worrying about happening in your life, no dramas to actually create something worth worrying about.

I will not, tell yourself, use dramas as a way of making life seem meaningful and interesting. I will just go and actually do something meaningful and interesting instead.

No more "hero" dramas and no more "victim" dramas. No more "too much" dramas, and no more "not enough" dramas. No more "you hate me" or "I hate you" dramas. No more dramas about the sad, sorry past, and no more dramas about the big, scary future. No more "my life is crap, and yours is so much better" dramas. We all have so much to be grateful for.

No more dramas. No more sending all that energy down a hole. No more head-miles on things that can't be changed. No more choosing, then choosing, then choosing again, and then forgetting where you started making choices and what the original problem even was you were trying to solve. No more talking about it on and on until it becomes something else it never was and didn't need to ever become.

Dramas are our way of giving ourselves something to deal with to avoid failing at our dreams. They're a distraction, a form of resistance against progress, because it's easier to never try than it is to try and fail. As someone with cancer, you have something significant happening to you right now, however don't use it as an excuse not to do and be what you were made for.

This is about who you are, not what you can't do.

No, no more dramas. No more for you. That's enough now, because time is short, and there's so much to be done. No more dramas. That's all over, forever. When you're ready to stop, we're ready too - ready to come and walk beside you, and with you, go anywhere you go and never leave your side. Come on - let's go.

No more excuses, distractions or resistance.

No more dramas.

Chapter 24
Funny Things People Say When You Have Cancer

What doesn't kill you makes you stronger.

Perhaps, but I've found however what doesn't kill you can still scare you pretty witless in the meantime. I don't want to be stronger one day - I want to feel better, now. Don't tell me one day - if I don't die - I'll be harder, meaner and braver. Just give me a hug instead.

There's always someone worse off than you.

I have cancer. That means I'm probably worse off than you are, at the very least. So that's actually true. I know what you mean though. However, I'm not the sort of person who becomes excited or inspired thinking about someone else who has something worse than cancer. If a person comforted by such thoughts exists, I think cancer is probably the least of their problems.

God is trying to teach you something.

You telling me this doesn't help. Even if it's true, which we have no way of knowing, you saying it still doesn't help. Even if I could know for certain God or the Universe was teaching me a lesson through my having cancer, and I knew what the lesson was, and I was actively participating in the learning of it, and even if I was about to graduate it with honors and a big old handshake from God Him-or-Herself, you telling me this still doesn't help. It really sounds like it might help, I appreciate that. It really does sound like a deep and spiritual thing to say, because we can't really understand God or the Universe or cancer, and lumping them all together in the same sentence seems like it would probably help, but it doesn't. Plus, if God really is trying to teach me something by giving me cancer, then God is probably a jerk, in which case I'm not going to particularly care about whatever it is He/She might be trying to teach me. So please, allow me to hold onto my childish fantasy about God being a Very Nice Deity who loves me and doesn't want to hurt me, which allows me to keep praying to Him/Her and ask Him if He'd/She'd mind helping me with my abject fear of dying of cancer. Thanks!

Things could be worse.

No, they fucking could not. Please leave now.

You don't look much like someone who has cancer.

You don't look much like a tactless jerk. Just goes to show.

Which breast was it in?

You know, despite what you may have been led to believe, not all cancer is breast cancer. So now please stop staring at my boobs.

My friend/cousin/uncle/neighbor had that, and they died.

Strangely, that information also isn't helpful.

Just pray, and God will heal you.

Tell you what - you pray, and I'll have chemo. *Bases covered*.

In case you're wondering, I'm being facetious. Even though people have quoted these cliché's to me, I've never said these things back again, unless you count in my head.

Look, the fact is, as hard as it is for us to have cancer, it's also really, really hard for the people around us. They don't know what to do or say, and the truth is, apart from producing copious amounts of both lasagna and cliché's, there isn't much they can do or say. Standing around while someone you care about suffers just sucks. People always, always mean well, even if the things they say don't make sense, aren't very helpful or offend us outright. Don't be angry. Just smile. Take the lasagna, and go punch a pillow. And as far as it's possible for you to do it, try and stay sweet, and keep your relationships one of those places cancer can't touch.

Chapter 25
When Dignity Wears A Size Smaller

A few months ago, I applied for a one-off government payment we were eligible for, which, unbeknown to me, invited an audit of past payments going back several years. After looking at my records, the social security department decided I was liable to repay a pension I received whilst my husband and I were separated for six months, so instead of getting a cheque in the mail for a few hundred dollars, I opened my mail to find a collection letter for several thousand dollars. Stunned, I called the agency for an explanation. The agency officer was patient, but firm. "You didn't abide by the child support agreement, which stipulates you must endeavor to recover by any means possible money owed to you in child support by the other party. You have to pay back your pension."

I asked to be allowed to appeal at a higher level.

Eventually, I was phoned up by another officer to discuss my appeal. I explained again how my husband and I were separated but he had no income for that time, so he couldn't pay child support, so in my mind there seemed no point in pursuing him. In fact, if she cared to check his records, she'd find he too was on benefits from the government, because he was too sick to work. I'd felt I didn't want to further exacerbate his condition by having a solicitor badger him for child support.

The officer was empathic, but unmoved. "You broke the agreement, you simply have to pay us back."

"Let me get this straight. So because my husband didn't pay me a couple of hundred dollars, you're going to make me pay you a few thousand?"

Up until then, I'd been trying to retain a semblance of dignity. My voice began to break. I started sobbing, still with the officer on the other end of the phone.

"Hold on, hold on. Just back up a little." She said. "Can you tell me, off the record, exactly what was going on around that time? I get the idea there's more to the story here than what you've told me."

I didn't want to tell her what happened. I felt it was all in the past, and I'd rather forget it all ever happened, but it seemed explaining the full story was the only way to make her understand.

"Well...I had cancer in 2003. I got better, but my husband didn't. He became an alcoholic, so I threw him out. We went to counseling, but while we were there he told me he didn't want to be married any more, but he agreed to go to rehab. While we were waiting for a place to come up in rehab, we lived under the same roof but fought every day. One day I followed him around the house yelling at him about how he'd let us all down and why couldn't he just man up and take responsibility when at one point he turned around with such desperation on his face - I'd never seen such despair in a human being before. In that moment, I knew if I didn't let him go, I'd come home one day and find him hanging from a tree.

"The short answer is I didn't try to collect child support because my alcoholic husband couldn't work, couldn't pay and was suicidal, and I was determined not to behave like a victim. I just wanted him to get better, and I wanted to get on with my life. "

It hurt having to tell her that story. I wanted to tell the story of our happy reconciliation, our present health and wholeness, how we paid up our debts and started fresh in a new town where nobody knew that victim story. In telling her about our unhappy past I felt like I was right back there with the pain and shame of being abandoned, broke and broken. We are not those people any more. But in an instant that was me again.

Thank God, she heard me. After hearing the truth about what happened, she sent my appeal up the chain and the agency cancelled the debt.

Victim stories are strange things. They can be painful, but they can also have utility when getting something you want or need. I get a plethora of victim stories every time I list something on Freecycle. It's awful for me, because then I have to decide who gets my washing machine - the single mum, the abandoned flat mate, the old-age pensioner? I don't want or like having that kind of power, and I don't enjoy having people tell me their problems in order to validate my generosity toward them.

Because I know how it feels.

When genuinely bad things happen to us like cancer, the way we are seen and see ourselves can change. We can find ourselves fighting others perceptions and projections, even if it's just in our own head. When I was staying at a hostel in Sydney near the hospital having radiotherapy, I remember walking down the hallway and passing the brass sponsor plaques beside each door. I hated those plaques. They were like little monuments to the slow, incremental death of my dignity. I didn't want to be reminded every morning I was a charity recipient. I was a charity recipient, and thank God I was, but any sense I was being pitied just repelled me. I didn't want to be seen or treated like I was less than simply by virtue of my circumstances.

When we have cancer, victim is a card we're handed whether we like it or not. It's up to us whether we play it. Sometimes, just like people who need washing machines or radiotherapy patients who need somewhere to stay in the big city, we have to play our card to access what we want or need. Sometimes we simply tear that card up and throw it away in disgust. Sometimes, as with me and the social security officer, the card is forced from our pocket and into plain view, and we have to use it even if we'd rather not.

You can only have so much control over how others see you, and the same amount of control over what actually happens to you. When you have cancer control can be diminished, but it could be you're prepared to let some go if you think it'll serve you. Some may pity you because it makes them feel superior, but this is rare. There can even be a degree of increased control, even power, in making yourself appear smaller. Regardless of how you play your victim card, the fact is nobody can ever remove your dignity from you by force. But you may find yourself buying it a size smaller, just for now.

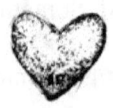

Chapter 26

Buy A Ticket

Cancer is a notorious hope destroyer.

Big hope. Little hope. Far off hope. Right here hope. All kinds of hope can come under threat when cancer comes near.

Cancer can seem like a roadblock between us and all the things we planned to do, hoped would happen and perhaps even took for granted.

So, what goes on here?

Well, it's the whole *death* thing. With cancer comes the very real possibility of our demise. This is often the first impact the cancer has - the realization we may have just encountered what could turn out to be the cause of our death.

And when you think you might be going to die in the foreseeable future, it kind of puts a damper on things.

Big things. Little things. Far off things. Right here things.

But we planned that trip for ten years.

But I thought I'd be here to see my daughter grow up.

But I just bought new shoes.

There's more than one way for cancer to kill you. If cancer takes away your dreams, desires and your hopes for the future, it's found a new way to do it. Don't let it.

Take care of your body first. Find out what you need to do about the cancer, and begin. Then take care of your hope.

One way to not let cancer kill your hope is to buy a ticket.

Buy a ticket. Talk about your plans for how life will be when cancer is gone. You may not know when this part of your life will end, but you can still think about how things will look and the things you'll do when it does.

Buy a ticket. A ticket to next week, next month or next year. Buy a ticket to your child's wedding, to the birth of your grandchild. Buy a ticket to your 25th anniversary, to your 40th, 50th, 60th, 70th and

80th birthday. Buy a ticket to your graduation, or to your son or daughters graduation.

Buy a ticket. Make a dream poster on a large piece of cardboard pasted all over with magazine clippings of people, things and places that inspire and excite you. Put it up where you can see it every day. Make your hope strong with daily exercise.

Buy a ticket. Literally. See the concert. Meet the author. Visit that place. See those sights. Definitely book the holiday.

Buy a ticket. For goodness sake, get the new shoes, even if you're afraid you'll never wear them out.

There is a difference between practicing hope however, and practicing denial. I once knew a woman diagnosed with late stage cancer who focused all her energy on getting out of hospital and over to a clinic on the other side of the country which promised to cure her. That's hope. However, she remained estranged from both her sons whom she refused to speak to, and also refused to hire a manager to run her business which struggled since the day she left to go to the doctor on her lunch break, and never came back. She died leaving an argument between the sons over her will and a business forced to close down. That's denial.

Buy a ticket. Create a stake in your future, in the currency that counts to you. Love travel? Plan the trip. All about family? See yourself with your grown children years from now. Imagine the outfit you'll wear to your sons wedding. See the shoes you'll wear. Write your speech.

I did. And stood up at my sons wedding and delivered it.

But what happens if that future never happens? What happens if cancer turns out to be the thing that ends your life?

The work we do on hope is never wasted. You'll be all the time investing in people you care about and in your relationships, and just as importantly in yourself. If you die, you'll leave a long, strong legacy of the evidence of who and what really mattered to you. And trust me, when you're not here any more, this is all the people who love you will want to know.

Buy a ticket. A ticket to your future. You're much, much more than what's happening to you right now. Resist the fear. Invest yourself in ways real and unreal in a life far above and way beyond cancer.

Chapter 27
What Really Matters

There's a scene in the movie City Slickers where Curly (played by Jack Palance) asks Mitch (Billy Crystal) if he knows what the secret of life is. Answering his own question, Curly holds up his pointer finger and says, "This one thing." Mitch, puzzled, asks Curly "But what's the one thing?" "That," says Curly cryptically, "is what you have to find out."

Late in 2003, I was told I was dying of cancer. I'd always thought being told you had cancer would probably be the worst part, but it wasn't like that for me. What worried me the most was the realization I hadn't worked out what *the one thing* was, not by a long shot.

Now, almost ten years later, I'm still working on it. I like to believe I'm closer than I was. My current operating theory runs like this: in order to work out what's really important - what *the one thing* is - it helps to know what isn't really important at all.

Here are a few things I've worked out are not really important to me.

Having a dust free house.

Being right every time, and making sure everyone knows it.

Knowing for certain whether there is a God or not, and whose side He or She is on.

Creating art or writing other people think is good.

Singing songs that other people think are good.

Winning.

Losing.

Having perky breasts.

My hair color.

My, or anyone else's, skin color.

Remembering who wronged me, when, and why.

Forgetting to apologize to those I've wronged.

Scatter cushions.

My parents mistakes.

My children's mistakes.

My own mistakes.

Succeeding at making others happy by failing to ever start trying to do what I suspect I was created to do.

Thinking the price for others' happiness is my misery.

Thinking the price for my happiness is others' misery.

Perfection.

Worrying about looking young.

Worrying about growing old.

Worrying what others think of me.

Worrying.

Winning. (I know I already said that but it's really not important.

Unless there's a gold medal at stake, and there usually isn't.)

Adapting my efforts to the opinions of critics.

Ignoring the advice of true friends, and very wise people.

Getting even.

Getting everything I think I have coming to me.

You getting what I think you have coming to you.

And there's more.

Isn't there, friend?

Could well be you'll work out what your *one thing* is, by clarifying what it isn't.

Chapter 28
Believe What God Says About You

Warning – Just need to let you know, I'm about to talk about God and in a way that may make you think I believe He exists. There's a reason for this – I do believe God exists. Besides, I need to talk to you about faith. The faith I'm about to talk to you about isn't necessarily to do with believing in God, but more to do with believing in you. If you don't believe in God, that's fine. Just know it takes as much faith to belief in yourself as it does just about anything else. I happen to think you may as well believe in God as anything, including yourself. I also happen to believe not just in God, but also that God believes in you.

Believe what God says about you.

Believing, in God or anything else for that matter, takes a step of faith - perhaps the very first one you've ever taken. Faith may be the last thing you feel capable of right now. But if you've ever read or heard someone's story and laughed or cried with it, or been moved or inspired by it, then you are capable of faith. It takes faith to believe, and to believe in someone's story, whether it really happened or is made up. If you've ever believed someone else's story as they told it to you, you have enough faith to believe in your own.

Believe what God says about you.

If you'll take this step of faith, then all the tangled, crumpled things will begin to unravel and unfold before you. You may begin to believe you can indeed let go when everything inside you screams to hold on. Letting go can feel like the last thing you want to do, but letting go is what you need to do to move beyond the here and now. There's a saying, "Let go, or be dragged." Can you remember how it feels to let go?

When you let go, you'll feel afraid, perhaps very afraid. But in surrender, you will begin to see everything afresh. What's been unclear and hidden from you will come into view. Your eyes will see horizons again. When was the last time you saw a horizon?

Believe what God says about you.

Faith is the first step, and will always be the first step toward healing, wholeness, health, freedom and future, whatever the outcome of this present challenge.

Yes, even if the worst possible case scenario seems or becomes inevitable, there's still room and scope for hope, healing and wholeness - in your soul and in your mind, in your relationships and in your religion. You can be healed, even if you don't survive this.

There are more ways than one for cancer to kill you. And there's more than one way for faith to heal you.

Believe what God says about you.

Don't be afraid. It's only one step.

The first step isn't a leap. A leap of faith may come later, after you've mastered the step. God knows you, and He knows where you are. He knows you're fragile right now. And He understands all you can cope with is one small step.

Believe what God says about you.

Listen. He's speaking.

"For I know the plans I have for you," says the Lord. "Plans for good and not for disaster, to give you a future and a hope. In those days when you pray, I will listen. If you look for me wholeheartedly, you will find me. I will be found by you," says the Lord. I will end your captivity and restore your fortunes. I will gather you out of the nations where I sent you and will bring you home again to your own land."*

You're far from home, far from where you want to be. This exile feels like hell, like punishment and retribution and spite. But it isn't those things. God hasn't punished you, but you have been captive to circumstances. He wants to make you free. He wants to make you whole, healed and free.

Your story now has a chapter about an exile and a captivity. It's not a perfect story any more. But there is a future and a hope in your story, still. God has written restoration and prosperity into your story. Don't believe what you see right now. Believe instead in the higher story.

Believe what God says about you.

*Jeremiah 29:11-14

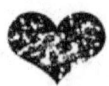

Chapter 29
Big Far Away, Where Hope Waits For Me

My eyes have deteriorated a lot over the last few months, mainly because I'm writing on a computer, and using social media far more than I once was. A friend of mine who also used to spend hours a day looking at a computer screen reckons after a couple of years living on a farm with wide skies and long views, his vision is improved amazingly. He says it's because he gets to look at things from a long way away all the time now. Tall trees. Horizons. The neighbors paddock. A child swimming across a dam. Gazing at faraway things has improved his physical sight, and, I venture, his imagination too.

As I look around our own compact home with security grills on every window, itself surrounded closely by other houses all of them shut in on themselves rather than opened up to the outside, it's no wonder my eyes are so tired. Everything in my world is right there, close-up, in my face. To see something far away, I need to get in my car and drive somewhere else - somewhere where the land meets the ocean, or the land meets the sky, or things grow which touch both the land and the sky. I wonder if I can retrain my eyes to see well again by looking into the distance more often.

When you have cancer, it's almost like the world closes in around you. You may even pull your walls in closer on purpose to give you something to hold you up, to make you feel safe. You may find it hard, even scary, to look too far into the future. Fear of not even having a future can force us to only look at what's right in front of us - the here and the now.

We may call this "living in the moment" – indeed, it sounds far more romantic than "What's the point of thinking about the future? I could be dead in a year."

In the cloister of the cancer world, our days can be reduced to a pattern of eating, drinking, sleeping, and being available for whatever needs to be done to get rid of cancer. It often doesn't feel much like "fighting cancer" - surely that would feel like doing something? We wait for results, we wait for appointments, we wait for side effects of treatment to kick in and abate again. We look at the walls of the inside of the rooms of our house, the insides of waiting rooms and clinics, the insides of cars and buses and taxis. We become dully familiar with places we never even noticed before - that weird space behind the toilet, the dust on the medicine cabinet shelf, the wrinkles on the inside of an elbow. There is no more wonder, serendipity or spontaneity. The air and the ground and the sea and the growing things must be kept away, and we from them, because they are wild with germs and dirt and chill and could make us even sicker. The walls grow higher. The colors grow greyer. The sky moves further away. Our vision for far away things begins to grow cloudy, whilst at the same time our ability to perceive the tiniest change in our body or immediate environment is heightened. Someone moved the soap. I can feel a lump. As night approaches, the sun edges closer to the horizon and the clouds recline before it, aroused into amazing purples and blushing orange and peach and gold...whilst we potter about our living room in our dressing gown and slippers, closing the window against the chill and our myopic eyes against the painful, boring day.

A gift we must give ourselves when we have cancer is the

opportunity to see things that are far away.

Things outside of us. Things towering over us, and running beneath us. Things lapping at our feet. Things dropping away before us. Things awesome and great, and small things. Things rushing by us, and things moving very slowly. Things we can only see when the earth turns. We need to see the sky and the stars and the horizon, the tallness and the depth and the proximity of things.

When you have cancer, take care to preserve your vision. Much like I need a break from this computer screen, and probably a break from my small house and neighborhood, you need a break from your small, closed-in world. Your vision - the way your mind, and your soul, sees the world - needs to spend some time out in open spaces, away from the cloister of a cancer experience. Imagination feeds hope, remember, and bigness, far-awayness, over-there-edness feeds your imagination with all the good and nourishing things it needs to stay alive.

Go outside. Go big far away. Look up at the stars. Count the sun-sparkles on the ocean. Run your hands through sand, dirt and stones. Find a place where there's a wide sky, and lay yourself beneath it. Throw up the blinds, and watch the wind cause chaos out there. Grow something where you can see it often and watch it. Throw something a long way away. Place space before you, and distance behind you. Hope is living as if you're heading now for everything you want and desire, as if it's just a matter of time - because one day you'll be there. You'll get there. Expand your long-distance vision further and further, and nurture your ability to see into your own future.

Your hope needs somewhere far away to wait for you.

Chapter 30
The Three Questions

The chapter you're about to read was the first one I wrote for this book, but there's no way it could come first. The thing is, what I'm about to say is what I'd like to say over and above just about everything you've read so far.

This is a conversation we may need to have - with ourselves, and with others - at some time or other. When things are going great in our lives, we pretty much have the luxury of avoiding stuff we don't want to talk or think about, much as we might hide a mess under the bed or food wrappers down the side of the couch. However, when something like cancer comes along, other things in our life often need to move around to make room. And when we start moving things around, our no-go zones become exposed to the wide, blue heavens and all God's children too. *Oh my God*, we cringe, *there's all that stuff I just couldn't face, didn't get around to, don't want to think about.*

Well, honey, guess what? You need to think about it now.

For an awful lot of people, thinking about dying is stuffed way, way under the bed. The plan generally is to deal with it quickly at the last possible moment. I wonder - would you recognize that last possible moment if you saw it coming?

These kinds of conversations are very hard to have. Nobody teaches us how to do it. Generally, in our culture, we don't even talk about death for goodness sake, even though we all die. Much of our dealing with dying is about pretending it isn't happening and wishing it wouldn't right up until it becomes inevitable. This isn't very helpful. We probably need to start talking about it way before then.

People don't like to talk about dying because death and dying is considered to be very, very bad, and to be avoided at all costs. Hello - of course, it is. Death is bad, obviously sad, and can also be tragic and untimely and unfair. But our refusal to even speak about death as being a part of life perpetuates the belief that all death is intrinsically bad, as in *wrong*, and we mustn't ever talk about it. Not all death is wrong. I've learned that whilst dying is unavoidable, it is actually possible to have a relatively good death. Not everyone gets one, but I think it's in all our best interests to see that those who could possibly have one do so.

One way we can improve the kinds of deaths people have is by stopping talking about it as if all death is a failure.

I especially become angry when it's carelessly remarked "They lost their battle with cancer." What if, in their mind, they never fought cancer? If they didn't fight cancer, but rather journeyed through cancer right to it's end (remember, when we die of cancer, cancer dies too), would that really be so awful, so wrong?

A few years ago, I heard someone speak about what we might say to someone facing their own death. The suggestions offered were so simple and so powerful, I'm passing them on as perhaps how you might want to think about death and dying, or perhaps have a conversation with someone who has been diagnosed with cancer. I'm not in any way suggesting this will be easy. It couldn't possibly be. But it will be at the very least clarifying. Perhaps even liberating.

When someone is diagnosed with cancer, there are three questions to consider:

Is it my time to die?

If it isn't my time, am I prepared to do what's required to survive?

If this is my time, am I ready for that?

The answers to these questions may impact not just how you journey through cancer and treatment, but also the quality of your life, or your death, at the end of it.

You can see now why I didn't put this chapter right at the beginning.

Of all the things I learned whilst I had cancer and since, learning how and when to have this conversation has been the most useful piece of information I've gleaned yet. I've had this talk with myself, and I've suggested it to others. I believe the conclusions we come to could very well be the only information we really need, whatever happens with the cancer. But that doesn't mean the conversation won't be confronting or uncomfortable.

We all want a good life, and a long one, but we don't always get one. Now, given my own health history, I don't know if I'll have a long life, but I sure as heck want a good one - and I also want a good death. I've known folks who didn't have a good death, and I believe this is as just as tragic as a short life or a wasted one. It may be time to move the couch and have a bit of a check underneath. Maybe the couch has already been moved, and you've relegated yourself to an upstairs closet to avoid facing the subject. If you've been avoiding it, I gently, loving suggest you don't avoid it, if at all possible.

Of the three questions I've suggested, you may only need to answer one, and knowing the answer to that one may make all the difference. This is not a formula, or a guarantee. It's simply a way for you to open up conversations between yourself and the folks you love, to help you recognize and acknowledge your priorities, your values and your resources.

I don't know what else to say, except it sucks we have to even think about this stuff whilst most people get to leave the couch where it is, and ignore the mess under the bed until much, much later. And I'm sorry about that. So much about having cancer is bad - not just inconvenient, unfair, and scary - but yep, plain old bad. I know you hate this. Me too. But what can we do? Well, the work these trying times require of us perhaps, and sometimes, that's enough.

Epilogue

So this is my last letter, the last thing my soul has to say to yours, at least for now. Thanks for allowing me to come with you on this part of your journey, it's been an honor, and I mean that most sincerely. When I was ill, I permitted very few to draw as close to me as you've allowed me to. Many well-written books given by well-intentioned friends hit the wall opposite my couch in my search for a soul sister or brother to sojourn with. If this one was thrown across the room, please know I understand, really, I do. I never meant to preach at you, or tell you what you were supposed to do or be as someone with cancer, but I do hope I've been able to help you glimpse a life beyond this experience, on the other side of cancer, whatever the outcome. You can be healed, you know, even if cancer never leaves, even if it stays with you, you can be well. There's no need to let cancer kill you in any of those other ways, don't give it that power, because that's the real tragedy - to die, while you live. Just remember - there's no way cancer gets out of this alive. You're always better, always stronger, always more than cancer. Your story matters, and cancer never, ever wins.

Love you always,

Jo

Read more about Jo Hilder

www.johilder.com

Other books by this author:

God, You Can Take My Mental Illness, Just Not The Part Where You Speak to Me

Things Not To Say To Someone Who Has Cancer

Available via www.johilder.com

and via Amazon and Amazon for Kindle

www.ingramcontent.com/pod-product-compliance
Lightning Source LLC
LaVergne TN
LVHW051603070426
835507LV00021B/2735